T0134925

Sleep Disorders in Pediatric Dentistry

Edmund Liem

Editor

Sleep Disorders in Pediatric Dentistry

Clinical Guide on Diagnosis
and Management

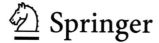 Springer

Editor
Edmund Liem
Vancouver TMJ & Sleep Therapy Centre
Burnaby, BC
Canada

ISBN 978-3-030-13271-2   ISBN 978-3-030-13269-9   (eBook)
https://doi.org/10.1007/978-3-030-13269-9

This Springer imprint is published by the registered company Springer Nature Switzerland AG
The registered company address is: Gewerbestrasse 11, 6330 Cham, Switzerland

Preface

Our world has been always in a constant change; things we used to do only 10 or 20 years ago could be obsolete, proven wrong, or replaced with new ideas. This applies to so many things, and the medical and dental world is no exception into this. This fast pace of change has implication to any profession, and without any doubt, every dentist has experienced this in his or her career.

Dentistry as it was taught 20 or more years ago was more conventional; it was considered as a separate discipline that only borders medicine. Dentistry is still taught as a profession for people with extreme good manual dexterity; most dentist can remember the dental school admission requirement of sculpting a soap bar. More and more emphasis is given to other qualities like:

- A desire to learn: Having a willingness to learn new things and a desire to improve your skills is a great trait. This is the best way to cope with constant change.
- Good problem-solving skills: Problem-solving skills are an essential trait for a dentist. Not every patient will have a dental/medical problem with a clear-cut solution. Sometimes a dentist needs to think outside the box in order to determine the best treatment approach for the patient.

Becoming a dentist takes an interest in science and a desire to help people.

Dentistry slowly becomes an important partner in healthcare; we have seen publications of correlations of the common gingivitis and heart disease [1]. Oral healthcare professionals can identify patients who are unaware of their risk of developing serious complications as a result of cardiovascular disease and who are in need of medical intervention.

We have seen publications about the value of early detection of oral cancer [2]. The prevention of oral cancer and its associated morbidity and mortality hinges upon the early detection of neoplastic lesions.

The oral cavity is an important anatomical location with a role in many critical physiologic processes, such as digestion, respiration, and speech. The mouth is frequently involved in conditions that affect the skin or other multi-organ diseases. In many instances, oral involvement precedes the appearance of other symptoms or lesions at other locations [3].

The latest trend is the involvement of dentistry in the management of obstructive sleep apnea [4]. The general dentist can play an important role in the recognition of signs and symptoms of patients with obstructive sleep apnea syndrome. Obstructive sleep apnea (OSA) is defined as the repetitive airway obstruction due to the collapse of the pharyngeal airway during sleep potentially causing partial or complete cessation of airflow for breathing. Although many suffer from symptoms of sleep apnea syndrome, most remain undiagnosed until significant problems occur, such as cardiopulmonary disease, neurologic dysfunction, and hypersomnolence. In recent years, sleep apnea has become a significant public health concern. Both medical and dental practitioners have become increasingly aware of sleep apnea. Early detection of this condition by the dental practitioner can lead to the prevention of comorbid diseases and improved quality of life for many patients.

General dentists are involved in the management of OSA of adults by providing alternative treatment with oral appliances (common acronyms: OAT, oral appliance therapy; MAD, mandibular advancement device; MAS, mandibular advancement splint). The gold standard for the treatment of OSA (adults and children) has been, and still is, the use of positive airway pressure (PAP) treatment. The immediate treatment outcome of the use of a PAP device is usually excellent; however, compliance is an issue. Adherence to positive airway pressure treatment for obstructive sleep apnea is a critical problem with adherence rates ranging from 30% to 60%. Poor adherence to PAP is widely recognized as a significant limiting factor in treating OSA, reducing the overall effectiveness of the treatment and leaving many OSA patients at heightened risk for comorbid conditions, impaired function, and quality of life [5]. Dentists who have received additional training can provide alternative treatment with OAT, and commonly the adherence rate is better than with PAP therapy [6].

OSA does not only affect adults; it does also affect children. The health consequences of OSA on adults are well documented [7]. There is now a wealth of information indicating that untreated obstructive sleep apnea is associated with an increased risk of fatal and nonfatal cardiovascular event, a higher propensity of sudden death during sleep, and a greater risk for stroke and all-cause mortality.

The health consequences for children with OSA are even more compelling. We have begun to understand that pediatric sleep disorders in general, and more particularly sleep-disordered breathing (SDB), can lead to substantial morbidities affecting the central nervous system (CNS), the cardiovascular and metabolic systems, and somatic growth, ultimately leading to reduced quality of current and future life. We have also monitored the altered behavior of children with OSA [8]. This can be confusing and can sometimes lead to a wrong diagnosis and treatment. Behavioral problems are prevalent in children with either mild SDB or OSA, and both groups of children show significant improvements in behavior after treatment. Research has also identified a link between sleep disorders and problematic and hyperactive behaviors and mood disturbances [9].

Charles Dickens has in 1836 described in his *The Pickwick Papers* a boy, called Joe, that has the characteristic of a person who suffers from sleep-disordered breathing [10]. Unknowingly, he described a child with pediatric SDB. This was the first description in the main literature about sleep-disordered breathing; for that reason, SDB is also initially known as the "Pickwickian syndrome."

The process of understanding pediatric sleep apnea is ongoing, and I am sure there is still a lot to be discovered. We already understand that pediatric sleep apnea has other dimensions than adult sleep apnea. Children are not just small people; strategies that apply to adults do not automatically apply to children. Side effects of OSA (adult) treatment are sometimes magnified when applied to children. As an example, we see that the compression forces of the mask of a PAP device limit the craniofacial growth of the child, potentially making the craniofacial structure more unfavorable for a normal (nasal) breathing.

There was a pilot study [11] with the pediatric application of MAD (oral appliances) that was designed for adults; after the initial promising results, we have not seen any further publications. One can only guess why this study has been terminated.

The most common cause of pediatric OSA is the enlargement of lymphoid tissue: adenoids and lingual tonsils. The enlargement of these tissues can create a structural blockage of the upper airway and higher airflow resistance. The most common treatment is the surgical removal of these tissues. Not enough attention is given why in the first place these tissues are hypertrophied; alternative management and understanding of these tissues will be researched in the coming years. Most importantly is that we need to develop a strategy to avoid adenotonsillar hypertrophy in the first place.

Quite commonly, children that are diagnosed with OSA do have a dysfunction in the way they breathe, speak, eat, and drink. Quite often, the children have an impaired nasal breathing leading to mouth breathing. A dysfunctional orofacial system is one of the causes of disturbed craniofacial growth and teeth crowding. A correction or, even better, reeducation of these functions has been shown in the literature as an effective (co-)treatment of pediatric OSA [12]. Current literature demonstrates that myofunctional therapy decreases apnea-hypopnea index by approximately 50% in adults and 62% in children! Myofunctional therapy could serve as an adjunct to other obstructive sleep apnea treatments.

The most promising treatment option of treatment of pediatric OSA is currently dentofacial orthopedic and orthodontics. This option has the ability to correct structural issues to improve nasal and pharyngeal airways. This allows to normalize structures so the orofacial complex can function how they should function. There are many publications [13–15] that report reduction of the apnea-hypopnea index after the expansion of the palate through rapid palatal expansion (RPE). It is believed that palatal expansion increases the palatal tongue space and nasal airway and facilitates nasal breathing.

In cases where there is a midfacial deficiency, a combination of palatal expansion with the use of a reverse pull headgear (protraction headgear) seems to have very good results [16].

One of the unknown and underestimated facts is that dentistry is in the best position to recognize the signs and symptoms of pediatric sleep apnea; dentists see children from a young age (2 years and up) on a scheduled regular base; they do inspect the orofacial region, and they could detect or recognize any signs or symptoms that could be related to pediatric sleep disorders. Dentists will also be able to observe the behavior and mood; this could sometimes be a sign of a pediatric sleep disorder.

However, at this time, there is a lack of awareness and education about this very important topic, and this book is one of the contributions to correct that void.

Burnaby, BC, Canada   Edmund Liem

References

1. http://www.ncbi.nlm.nih.gov/pmc/articles/PMC3100856/
2. http://www.ncbi.nlm.nih.gov/pubmed/9089529
3. http://emedicine.medscape.com/article/1081029-overview
4. http://www.ncbi.nlm.nih.gov/pubmed/24192732
5. http://www.ncbi.nlm.nih.gov/pmc/articles/PMC2972705/
6. http://www.ncbi.nlm.nih.gov/pmc/articles/PMC1794626/
7. http://www.ncbi.nlm.nih.gov/pmc/articles/PMC2645248/
8. http://www.ncbi.nlm.nih.gov/pubmed/17667138
9. http://journals.lww.com/co-pulmonarymedicine/Abstract/2007/11000/Neurocognitive_and_behavioral_morbidity_in.7.aspx
10. http://www.charlesdickensinfo.com/novels/pickwick-papers/the-pickwick-papers-and-sleep-apnea-charles-dickens/
11. http://news.ubc.ca/2009/02/05/archive-ubcreports-2009-09feb05-apnea/
12. http://www.ncbi.nlm.nih.gov/pubmed/25348130
13. http://www.ncbi.nlm.nih.gov/pmc/articles/PMC3004500/
14. https://www.researchgate.net/publication/261763395_The_impact_of_rapid_palatal_expansion_on_children's_general_health_A_literature_review
15. http://www.ncbi.nlm.nih.gov/pubmed/21437777
16. http://www.jdsm.org/ViewArticle.aspx?pid=30401

Acknowledgments

My most sincere appreciation is to my parents who have guided me throughout my life. Without their guidance and encouragements, I would never be in the position where I am now.

This book is dedicated to them.

I wish to thank the many friends (dental colleagues and assisting staff) I have met on my 40+ year journey through the never-ending development of my professional side; they have shared comraderies, knowledge, and passion for the best health outcome of the patients who have trusted us. We have started in dentistry with blinders on our eyes and after many years, slowly our vision has widened, and we are now amazed how much interaction and participation we can have in the care of the total health of our patients.

It is impossible to list everybody who has influenced me on my journey, so I will name the 4 most influential persons in my professional career as a dentist:

- Dr. John Witzig whose passion sparks me to explore the world of functional orthodontics
- Dr. Brock Rondeau who gave me a solid foundation in orthodontics
- Dr. John Mew who gave me the understanding of the importance of "oral posture"
- Dr. Steven Olmos who taught me the connection of TMD and OSA

I thank my 7 other siblings (2 of them are also dentists) for encouraging me in my profession.

Last but not least, I thank all the coauthors of this book; without their willingness to share knowledge and their hard work, this book would never have seen the daylight.

Edmund Liem

Contents

Contributors

Kevin L. Boyd, DDS, MS Lurie Children's Hospital, Chicago, IL, USA
Private practice, Dentistry for Children, Chicago, IL, USA

Osman S. Ipsiroglu, MD Department of Paediatrics, Faculty of Medicine, University of British Columbia, Vancouver, BC, Canada
H-Behaviours Research Lab [Previously Sleep/Wake-Behaviour Research Lab], BC Children's Hospital Research Institute, University of British Columbia, Vancouver, BC, Canada

Edmund Liem, DDS Vancouver TMJ & Sleep Therapy Centre, Burnaby, BC, Canada

Edmund A. Lipskis, DDS, MS The Centre for Integrative Orthodontics, St. Charles, IL, USA

Martha Macaluso, RDH Academy of Orofacial Myofunctional Therapy, Pacific Palisades, CA, USA
New York University College of Dentistry, New York, NY, USA

Ruth Marsiliani, RDH Academy of Orofacial Myofunctional Therapy, Pacific Palisades, CA, USA
New York University College of Dentistry, New York, NY, USA
The City University of New York, New York City College of Technology, Brooklyn, NY, USA

Joy L. Moeller, RDH Academy of Orofacial Myofunctional Therapy, Pacific Palisades, CA, USA

German O. Ramirez-Yañez, DDS, MS Private Practice, Aurora Kids Dentistry, Aurora, ON, Canada

Barry Raphael, DDS Raphael Center for Integrative Orthodontics, Clinton, NJ, USA

Manisha Budhdeo Witmans, MD University of Alberta, Edmonton, AB, Canada

Seng-Mun (Simon) Wong, DDS Private Practice, Melbourne, VIC, Australia
Orthotropics Module, Department of Orthodontics, University of Valencia, Valencia, Spain

Obstructive Sleep Apnea Syndrome

1

Manisha Budhdeo Witmans

1.1 Introduction

Sleep is a basic physiological need, and humans spend about one third of their lives sleeping. Sleep architecture is composed of two basic types of sleep called rapid eye movement (REM) sleep and non-REM (NREM) sleep. NREM sleep can be further subdivided into stages N1, N2, and N3, which make up different portions of the night that the individual spends sleeping. The amount of each stage can change on the basis of the person's age. Less is known about gender differences in sleep. The different sleep stages are characterized by different electroencephalogram patterns and electro-oculography patterns. NREM sleep makes up 75% of the night (5% is stage N1 sleep, 45–55% is stage N2 sleep, and about 25% is stage N3 sleep), while REM sleep accounts for the remaining 25% [1]. In contrast to children and adults, infants spend almost 50% of the time in REM sleep, and as much as 80% of sleep is spent in REM sleep in premature infants. Physiologically, humans are most vulnerable to perturbations in breathing during REM sleep, thus often classified as sleep-related breathing disorders when there are associated disturbances in gas exchange. The primary sleep disorder associated with breathing abnormalities in REM sleep is obstructive sleep apnea (OSA). Different names are used to describe the spectrum of this disorder and may include upper airway resistance syndrome, sleep apnea, obstructive apnea, sleep-disordered breathing, and obstructive sleep apnea hypopnea syndrome. This form of sleep-disordered breathing is different from central sleep apnea and hypoventilation, which are related to other pathophysiological mechanisms and involve different treatment options. The reader is encouraged to read the *International Classification of Sleep Disorders* (3rd Edition) for more comprehensive discussion and explanations about the various sleep-related breathing disorders. The focus of the following discussion will be relevant to obstructive sleep apnea. This is arguably a very important disorder in sleep medicine, as it has many

M. B. Witmans (✉)
University of Alberta, Edmonton, AB, Canada

© Springer Nature Switzerland AG 2019
E. Liem (ed.), *Sleep Disorders in Pediatric Dentistry*,
https://doi.org/10.1007/978-3-030-13269-9_1

serious consequences for the affected individuals, including increased morbidity and mortality and for society in general as its impact affects performance, vigilance, and optimal functioning. Unfortunately, at this time, although there are treatment options that may help manage the resulting symptoms and prevent complications, we are certainly nowhere near the point of lifelong cure. The treatment may alleviate or reduce symptoms and sequelae for a period of time; age is a risk factor for persistence or recurrence of the disorder. However, we remain hopeful that advances in science and technology will improve the management of sleep apnea and enable us to develop more customized and individual specific treatment options.

1.2   History

Obstructive sleep apnea was initially reported in the 1970s. It has become increasingly prevalent and is a significant public health problem. Descriptions of OSA in the lay literature can be traced back to Shakespeare, as well as the famous character Joe from *The Pickwick Papers*, the Charles Dickens novel. Use of the term Pickwickian syndrome is discouraged because this term is not only used to describe obstructive sleep apnea but also has been used to describe individuals with obesity hypoventilation syndrome. In the medical literature, Dr. John Cheyne was the first person to describe sleep-disordered breathing associated with heart failure and an irregular breathing pattern during sleep [2]. Cases were slowly reported over time until the mid-twentieth century, when the problem became widely recognized, and its consequences extend to every sphere of medicine. Obesity was thought to be the primary factor in the development of sleep apnea, until the 1970s, when Drs. Dement and Guilleminault showed that sleep apnea could occur in thin individuals [1]. They were instrumental in establishing the field of sleep medicine and first described OSA in children in 1976 [1]. Since then, the field has expanded exponentially to become a subspecialized field of medicine, rooted in several disciplines, including respirology, neurology, psychiatry, psychology, pediatrics, otolaryngology, internal medicine, cardiology, anesthesia, and dentistry.

Obstructive sleep apnea is a disorder characterized by recurrent episodes of partial upper airway obstruction (hypopnea) or complete upper airway obstruction (apnea) during sleep, despite respiratory efforts, and it results in sleep disruption, usually an arousal, and ventilatory instability [3] (drops in oxygen saturation, and swings in blood pressure during the apneic episodes). The Task Force of the *International Classification of Sleep Disorders* (3rd Edition) has defined obstructive sleep apnea in children and adults separately, particularly because of the differences in the diagnostic criteria noted below. The spectrum of disordered breathing during sleep can range from snoring to frank OSA with its associated consequences. Snoring is more prevalent in children and adults compared to OSA, with rate estimates ranging from 17% to 33% in men versus 7–19% in women (Principles and Practice of Sleep Medicine). OSA associated with daytime sleepiness affects 3–7% of adult men and 2–5% of adult women [1]. Depending on the criterion used, the lowest estimates suggest 4% prevalence in males and 2% prevalence in females. A recent systematic review determined the prevalence rates to be widely variable in adults, based on the threshold for defining sleep apnea, and estimated rates as high as 49%! In some older age groups, the estimates were higher than 80% [4]. In children the prevalence rates of OSA vary from 1% to 5%, depending on the diagnostic criteria used to define OSA. The disease defining quantitative parameter used to calculate the frequency and severity of airflow obstruction is called the apnea–hypopnea index (AHI) (Table 1.1), measured during overnight polysomnography (PSG). The American Academy of Sleep Medicine (AASM) has classified the severity of sleep apnea on the basis of cutoffs for apnea/hypopnea. Mild, moderate, and severe OSA are classified as ≥ 5, ≥ 15, and ≥ 30 events per hour, respectively. OSA-related symptoms include excessive daytime sleepiness, morning headaches, behavioral mood problems, insomnia, and identified comorbidities such as hypertension. The challenge of this definition is that using this as the only indicator of disease is that it fails to provide information regarding the physiological and/or functional impact of this disorder on affected individuals. Various candidate genes such as TNFa have been linked to phenotypes of OSA and are being evaluated.

What is not understood with absolute certainty is the threshold of change from benign snoring to OSA along the continuum of breathing during sleep. Snoring may certainly be disruptive to a bed partner or the affected individual but does not result in any reportable consequences. In contrast, it is arguable that any snoring reflects airflow limitation in the airway, and any resulting consequences may not be appreciated until the severity of the problem is significant enough to affect the bed partner or to result in sleepiness, daytime impairment, and/or cardiovascular consequences.

Table 1.1 Types of events associated with obstructive sleep apnea, according to the American Academy of Sleep Medicine (*AASM*) [5] scoring manual in adults. In children, the same definitions apply but the duration is for greater than or equal to 2 breaths and not 10 seconds. Children 13–18 can be scored using adult criteria.

Obstructive apnea: Decrease in the peak airflow signal excursion by 90% of the pre-event baseline for 10 s with continued or increased respiratory effort throughout the entire period of absent airflow

Hypopnea: Decrease in the peak airflow signal excursion by 30% of the pre-event baseline for 10 s with associated arousal or 3% oxygen desaturation with any one of the following: snoring, increased inspiratory flattening of the airflow signal, or associated thoracoabdominal paradox

Central apnea: Decrease in the peak airflow signal excursion by 90% of the pre-event baseline for 10 s with absent respiratory effort throughout the entire period of absent airflow

Central hypopnea: Decrease in the peak airflow signal excursion by 30% of the pre-event baseline for 10 s with associated arousal or 3% oxygen desaturation with none of the following: snoring, increased inspiratory flattening of the airflow signal, or associated thoracoabdominal paradox

Hypoventilation: Increase in the arterial PCO_2 to a value 55 mmHg for 10 min or an increase in arterial PCO_2 by 10 mmHg from the awake baseline to a value >50 mmHg for 10 min. In children, this is defined as hypercapnia, or increased $PCO_2 > 50$ mmHg for at least 25% of the total sleep time.

PCO₂ partial pressure of carbon dioxide

In fact, snoring alone has been associated with excessive daytime sleepiness, and those who snore tend to have a higher Epworth sleepiness score (ESS) >10 [6]. In children, snoring has been associated with poorer executive function. As in other disorders, many of the origins of adult sleep apnea may stem from infancy or childhood. Children with OSA have been found to have elevated blood pressure 10–15 mmHg higher than nonsnoring controls during sleep, irrespective of the severity of the sleep apnea [7]. OSA is a highly prevalent and serious chronic disease with significant morbidity and mortality and with increasing prevalence worldwide [8]. If it does indeed start in childhood, this behooves us to address the problem early and comprehensively.

1.3   Pathogenesis

Obstructive sleep apnea occurs because there is a lack of adequate compensation to maintain an open airway when the normal reduction in pharyngeal dilator muscle activity is superimposed on a narrowed airway with increased collapsibility [9]. A Starling resistor model is used to explain the human pharyngeal airway during sleep [10]. However, the inspiratory flow decreases with increasing effort which is called negative effort dependence, rather than being fixed as predicted by the Starling model. Wellman and colleagues have shown that the resistance in the upper airway can vary considerably in patients with sleep apnea and in turn influence downstream narrowing as well [11]. Although the pathogenesis of OSA has not been conclusively determined, certain factors have been identified that are attributable to obstructive sleep apnea. (1) Pharyngeal anatomy and collapsibility determine the critical closing pressure, which is the pressure at which the airway will narrow or close as described above and its inherent variability within individuals. This has been shown to be less negative, meaning more collapsible, in children and adults with sleep apnea. (2) Ventilatory control system gain or loop gain, which is the responsivity of the system to deal with perturbations in respiratory control. Therefore, a high loop gain will promote apneas as a response to the initial disturbance because of overcompensation, whereas a low loop gain will reduce the perturbations in breathing [12]. (3) The ability of the airway to dilate or stiffen in response to an increase in ventilatory drive. (4) Arousal threshold is the point at which an individual may respond to the apnea and the associated perturbations with a cortical arousal to an apnea. (5) Fluid shift which refers to the increased volume of venous fluid and/or upper airway mucosal fluid may contribute to the decreased surface area and increased resistance during sleep, which may decrease the volume of the airway during sleep [13]. Elegant work by Marcus and colleagues in children have shown that children with obstructive sleep apnea have impaired two-point discrimination in the tongue and palate compared to healthy controls [14]. They also showed that the palate is not affected as it is in adults when using vibration perception as a measurement in small number of control with sleep apnea [15]. Taken together, this has implications for selecting specific treatment targets for children and adults with sleep apnea depending on how the upper airway is affected during sleep. There have been developments in the last several years to try and phenotype adults in order to discern best treatment options for the sleep apnea. However, this is difficult in children for many reasons.

1.4   Risk Factors

It was assumed that OSA is a disorder in adults only. However, this is not the case, because OSA can affect any individual from cradle to grave, and we are learning that the syndrome involving obstructive sleep apnea includes signs and symptoms resulting from partial or complete upper airway obstruction leading to arousals, sleep fragmentation, hypoxemia, hypercapnia, and blood pressure perturbations during sleep [16]. The genetic predisposition towards OSA is largely inherited based on racial studies, chromosomal mapping, familial studies, and twin studies. About 35–40% of the variance in the pathogenesis for OSA can be attributed to genetic factors. The genetic factors may be associated with body fat distribution, craniofacial structure, and neurophysiological control of the upper airway, and central regulation of breathing that may be affected. The interaction of these factors and possible environmental factors may result in the wide range of effects that are seen with OSA syndrome. The definitions and how the OSA was measured in various studies may account for the great variances found among the studies. Nevertheless, genetic underpinnings are an important consideration and may affect the likelihood of comorbidities as well. The strongest risk factors for OSA are obesity and male gender [17]. Although obesity increases the risk of sleep apnea about 10–14 fold, it accounts for about 30–50% of the variance suggesting involvement of other factors. There are genetic overlaps between the factors that mitigate obesity and OSA. Increasing age is also a risk factor for increased airway collapsibility. In addition, craniofacial structure involving the hard and soft tissue features of the upper airway is also genetically determined. Various features such as macroglossia, retrognathia, micrognathia, and type II malocclusion, elongated soft palate, and inferior displacement of the hyoid have been implicated. Ventilatory control patterns may also play a role in influencing breathing during sleep but also the airway collapsibility. Abnormal ventilatory responses have been implicated and may shed some light on why some individuals are more susceptible than others. Further impact of genes involving sleep and circadian rhythm may also further influence the phenotype of sleep apnea, and increasing age increases the likelihood of sleep apnea. Risk factors for OSA include a body mass index (BMI) $\geq$ 35 kg/m^2, advancing age, male gender, structural factors (craniofacial abnormalities, hypotonia as in all individuals with Down syndrome, nasal obstruction, and an increased neck circumference), ethnicity, family history, cigarette smoking/exposure to environmental tobacco smoke (in children), lower socioeconomic status, and a history of prematurity [1]. Endocrine-related disorders such as hypothyroidism and acromegaly are also risk factors for OSA. OSA is more common is individuals with certain neurological disorders affecting the muscles such as myotonic dystrophy. OSA severity is also likely affected by alcohol consumption [18] and/or use of sedative medication before sleep onset. Conditions associated with OSA are listed in Table 1.2.

Male sex is certainly an important risk factor in adults, in that the male-to-female ratio of the reported prevalence is 2-3:1, but this has not been reported in children, as boys and girls are equally affected. Women tend to have an increased risk of OSA after menopause, decreasing the disparity in gender. The presentation in women like cardiovascular disease also tends to be different. Obesity is strongly linked with OSA. An increase in body weight of 10% has been associated with a sixfold greater risk of developing OSA, in comparison with healthy weight [19, 20]. Nasal congestion, resulting in airflow obstruction, has also been linked to obstructive sleep apnea, and more severe OSA is linked to individuals with allergies, compared with nonallergic individuals [21–23]. Finally, certain genetic craniofacial conditions—such as Apert, Crouzon, Marfan, Pierre Robin, and Down syndromes—are also associated with a higher prevalence of OSA [24].

1.5   Clinical Features

Obstructive sleep apnea is a relatively common but underdiagnosed disease with significant sequelae. The symptom cluster is often brought to light because snoring during sleep is either disruptive to the bed partner or results in daytime impairment for the affected individual (excessive daytime sleepiness, insomnia from fragmented night time, or associated conditions or comorbidities that become apparent, such as hypertension). Since the onset can be insidious and can occur at any age, all health care providers should have a low threshold for screening for OSA. Dentists are ideally positioned to implement screening for OSA in their practice. Common presenting features of OSA include loud snoring, choking, gasping, increased work of breathing during sleep, and pauses in breathing in adults. Other reported symptoms may include gastroesophageal reflux, mood disturbance, and erectile dysfunction. In children, similar symptoms may occur, but children tend to have more partial airflow obstruction with increased work of breathing and not frank apneas as adults. The compliant chest wall makes them more vulnerable to paradoxical

Table 1.2 Associations and comorbidities

Metabolic dysregulation including type 2 diabetes

Hypertension

Congestive heart failure, atrial fibrillation, ischemic heart disease, and presence of OSA may further exacerbate underlying conditions

Pregnancy

Headache, cerebrovascular disease, or stroke

Depression

Respiratory disease (asthma, chronic obstructive pulmonary disease, pulmonary hypertension, pulmonary fibrosis) and the presence of OSA may further exacerbate underlying conditions

Gastroesophageal reflux disease

breathing, particularly in REM sleep. Children who have muscle weakness, low tone, or hypermobility syndromes may not snore, but may present with obstructive hypoventilation. The children may sleep in unusual positions to maintain airway patency. The affected individual may be unaware of the symptoms, but concerns may be brought to light by the bed partner or a parent. Associated symptoms can range from insomnia to fragmented sleep, nonrestorative sleep, and morning headaches. Nocturia and secondary enuresis have also been linked to OSA. This sleep fragmentation resulting from arousals secondary to OSA may present as excessive daytime sleepiness, hyperactivity, moodiness, or irritability or even as attention and behavior issues in children. Academic performance may be affected including executive functioning and working memory. Excessive sleepiness may be present in older children and adolescents but less commonly noted in children. The OSA features may also be associated with other sleep disorders because of OSA-induced arousals resulting in parasomnias (confusional arousals, sleepwalking, night terrors) or REM behavior disorder. There may be comorbid seizure disorder, which may either be exacerbated by sleep apnea or the sleep apnea may result in seizures. Parents may cosleep with their children out of concern or worry because of the severity of apneas or to be present to stimulate the child to breathe.

Features that could increase the suspicion of sleep apnea on physical examination for development of OSA include craniofacial and upper airway abnormalities, malocclusion, obesity, and increased neck circumference in adults. Airway dimensions are often graded clinically using the Mallampati classification to objectively state the airway relationship, which ranges from class I (an easily viewed airway) to class IV (inability to view the posterior pharynx because of the position of the tongue and palate). Higher grades suggest a more crowded airway and thus an increased risk of sleep apnea. In children, adenotonsillar hypertrophy is the most common reason in preschool children and obesity in adolescence. The tonsil size is similarly graded from grade 0 to grade 4, which denotes kissing tonsils. In children, the grade of the tonsils can be helpful but do not always correlate with the severity of the symptom complex or the severity of the apnea hypopnea index. Other factors in children can be related to the conditions that involve craniofacial abnormalities such as cleft palate, and mucopolysaccharidoses.

1.6 The United Airway of Inflammation: Rhinitis, Asthma, and Sleep Apnea. Causal or Association?

It is apparent that OSA is a disorder resulting in systemic inflammation, as evidenced by the plethora of evidence linking sleep apnea, obesity, and cardiovascular outcomes. Therefore, any inflammatory condition could certainly contribute to the severity of OSA. Asthma is one of the most prevalent chronic diseases in children. The prevalence of OSA and asthma have increased in the last decade. They share common inflammatory mediators such as cysteinyl leukotrienes. Studies in both children and adults have shown that asthma increases the likelihood of OSA and sleep apnea can make asthma management more difficult [25–28]. In fact,

Bhattacharjee evaluated asthma outcomes based on a database of 13,506 children with asthma who underwent an adenotonsillectomy. Asthma outcomes were compared in the year preceding tonsillectomy versus after adenotonsillectomy. In addition, 27,012 age, sex, and geographically matched children with asthma without adenotonsillectomy were included to include asthma outcomes in children without known OSA. In the children who underwent the adenotonsillectomy with OSA and asthma, the adenotonsillectomy was associated with significant reductions in acute asthma exacerbations (30.2%), acute status asthmaticus episodes (37.9%), asthma-related emergency room visits (25.6%), and asthma-related hospitalizations (35.8%). Furthermore, adenotonsillectomy was associated with significant reductions in most asthma prescription refills, including bronchodilators (16.7%), inhaled corticosteroids (21.5%), LTRA (13.4%), and systemic corticosteroids (23.7%) [29]. It is clear that the two chronic diseases are related but what is still not established is if there is causality implying that one leads to the other [30]. Rhinitis and asthma are linked, and in turn, they are associated with OSA and can overlap with reflux. Obesity further complicates these interrelationships in that obesity itself is a risk factor for both asthma and OSA. Factors linking asthma, obesity, and sleep apnea may include mechanical factors and activation of the inflammatory cascade, which is exacerbated by hypoxemia. Gastroesophageal reflux disease has also been linked to OSA. Although adenotonsillar hypertrophy is the most commonly cited etiology, the underlying reason for the lymphoid hyperplasia may be related to atopic disease or systemic inflammation in general and lymphoid tissue such as lingual tonsils have also been reported. Some of the inflammation may be related to common cellular mechanisms. Therefore, other conditions mediating inflammation such as gastroesophageal reflux, or atopic disease such as food allergy, or eosinophilic esophagitis may also further exacerbate inflammation. Most recently, inflammation related to celiac disease has also been linked to OSA symptoms in children and a gluten-free diet led to resolution of symptoms [31]. These associations therefore suggest that the pathophysiological processes resulting in symptoms can be quite complex and multifactorial. any health, any health professionals, particularly dentists, are in the ideal position to screen for sleep-disordered breathing and be involved in the management of the airway with the other specialists.

1.7   Sequelae Associated with Obstructive Sleep Apnea

Dr. David Gozal was one of the first people to present strong evidence that OSA affects academic performance in children. He evaluated schoolchildren in grade 1 for OSA and showed that those who underwent an adenotonsillectomy for OSA had a substantial improvement in their academic performance in grade 2, equivalent to an intelligence quotient (IQ) increase of 10 points [32]. Gozal and Pope evaluated this hypothesis further, linking poor academic performance to associated snoring. They asked if adolescents had snored during childhood and had undergone an adenotonsillectomy, and they found that 13% of poorly performing adolescents had snored loudly, versus only 5% of high-performance adolescents. In addition, 3% had undergone an adenotonsillectomy in infancy due to snoring, versus only 1% of the high performers [33]. These findings illustrate that OSA can result in long-lasting adverse cognitive consequences. Moreover, Dr. Ron Chervin showed that OSA led to hyperactive behavior in a pediatric population [34]. Since that study by Dr. Gozal, elegant research by his group and others have shown that obstructive sleep apnea is linked to sequelae in children across metabolic, cardiovascular, and neurobehavioral domains (Principles and Practice of Sleep Medicine).

Clinicians often ask how much snoring is too much and what differentiates persistent versus transient snorers. It appears that there is a difference. In one study the strongest predictors of persistence of snoring were lower socioeconomic status and absence of breast feeding or a shorter duration of it, and persistent snorers had significantly higher rates of behavioral problems, particularly hyperactivity and depression [35]. These factors allude to the role of epigenetics in determination and persistence of airway obstruction. Ongoing work with genes and biomarkers will shed further light in this area.

Untreated sleep apnea is associated with hypertension, myocardial infarction, cardiac failure, stroke, cardiac dysrhythmias, increased risk of motor vehicle accidents, and sudden death. Furthermore, there is emerging evidence that neurocognitive abilities—including attention, working memory, and executive function—are also impaired in individuals with OSA. It is not only children with sleep apnea who have an increased risk of injury; adults with OSA are also more likely to have motor vehicle crashes from drowsy driving. The rising prevalence rates of obesity has also led to an increase in the prevalence of OSA. Data from the Wisconsin Cohort study showed that a 10% increase in body weight was associated with a sixfold increase in the development of OSA over a 4-year period and rise in AHI by 32% [36].

1.8 Why Is Pediatric Sleep Apnea Different from Adult Sleep Apnea?

Although, by definition, OSA is a condition that can occur along the continuum of the life-span—from cradle to grave—the nature, characteristics, and presentation of sleep-disordered breathing or sleep apnea differ between children and adults. Some basic developmental reasons why children are different from adults include a smaller airway, more fatigable muscles, less respiratory reserve, a more collapsible airway, and younger age [37]. There is limited evidence as to whether OSA in children is predictor of adult OSA.

Narrow nasal and nasopharyngeal airways, narrow dimensions of the maxilla, and positional or relative differences between the cranial base, maxilla, and mandible have been reported in both children and adults with nasopharyngeal obstruction related to adenoids using various techniques from acoustic rhinometry, cone beam CT, and lateral cephalograms and most recently dynamic MRI to assess the airway [38].

An interesting retrospective review recently showed that nasal obstruction related not only to adenoidal hypertrophy but also to a narrow nasal maxillary complex may contribute to OSA in adults [39]. The authors suggested that smaller dimensions related to the nasal maxillary complex in children with more severe nasal obstruction appeared to be continuous by age. This finding supports the notions that there are indeed childhood origins of adult OSA and that early intervention could potentially result in improved outcomes. This would be best accomplished by an interdisciplinary team, addressing different anatomical, neuromuscular, and skeletal relationships to optimize airway diameter stability.

1.9   Diagnosis

There is a spectrum of sleep-related breathing disorders. The most prevalent is OSA, affecting about 1–3% of children. The gold standard method for diagnosing OSA and sleep-disordered breathing is overnight laboratory PSG. However, this is a cumbersome, resource-intensive, and very specialized diagnostic procedure with limited access. There are ongoing efforts to develop more simplified, easily accessible tools with devices that include cardiorespiratory signals or, in some cases, just one or two recording channels, such as oximetry. Evidence has been established for the diagnostic utility of these ambulatory devices in comparison with that of PSG, particularly in severe OSA, in adults [40]. More recently, a randomized, controlled, multicenter trial has provided strong support for the role of ambulatory testing (or home sleep apnea testing) in the treatment and management of OSA. In fact, it showed that ambulatory devices were equally efficacious and more cost effective in managing symptoms in individuals with sleep apnea [41]. However, home sleep testing is contraindicated in individuals with heart failure, neuromuscular disease, significant chronic lung disease, or hypoxemia. In those individuals, an attended in-laboratory study is preferred. In contrast, there is limited evidence for home sleep apnea testing in children. Two small studies have shown that ambulatory studies can be used as a screening tool for OSA in the context of a more comprehensive clinical evaluation. For many years, oximetry has been used in Canada to screen for OSA in children [42, 43], and it is more easily accessible than laboratory PSG. Although there have been tremendous improvements in the technology used to diagnose OSA, the skills and instrumentation required make it a highly specialized service, which is readily available to only a few. There is also ongoing active research aimed at identifying OSA in children by using biomarkers or metabolites. Unfortunately, we are still years away from a simple and effective biomarker test for use in screening for OSA.

There is interest in identifying factors that are helpful for predicting the likelihood of the need for treatment of OSA and, more importantly, which children are ideal candidates for surgery. The children in the surgical treatment arm of the Childhood Adenotonsillectomy (CHAT) study were assessed to determine if PSG data or the Pediatric Sleep Questionnaire (PSQ) offered any predictive value for improvement related to obstructive sleep apnea syndrome (OSAS). At baseline, each 1–standard deviation (SD) increase in the baseline PSQ score was associated with an adjusted odds ratio that was approximately 3–4 times higher for behavioral morbidity, 2 times higher for reduced global quality of life, 6 times higher for reduced disease-specific quality of life, and 2 times higher for sleepiness. Higher baseline PSQ scores (denoting a greater symptom burden) also predicted postsurgical improvement in parent ratings of executive functioning, behavior, quality of life, and sleepiness. In contrast, baseline PSG data did not independently predict these morbidities or their postsurgical improvement. Neither PSQ nor PSG data were associated with objectively assessed executive dysfunction or improvement at follow-up [44]. What these data tell us is that the PSQ may be a good tool to use in an office setting to identify children at risk. The CHAT study data were also used to determine if any clinical parameters could predict OSAS severity in children. It was concluded that although a number of clinical parameters are associated with severity of OSA in children, none of the demographic variables, physical findings, nor questionnaire responses were able to predict OSA severity [45]. This implies that objective testing is essential for determining the severity of OSA in children and planning for perioperative care, but the PSG related variables in the CHAT study were not able to predict postoperative complications [46]. Explanations may include the limited hypoxemia criteria for inclusion in the study, the restricted age range of the children (5–9 years), the inclusion of relatively healthy children, and performance of the study at academic centers where the expertise of the attending clinical teams would likely be a confounder. In other studies, overnight pulse oximetry has been shown to be helpful in planning of perioperative care [47–50].

1.10 Treatment of Obstructive Sleep Apnea

The treatment of OSA is multifactorial, with the aim being to improve airway patency. Some of the interventions include limiting or omitting exposure to environmental tobacco smoke, particularly for children, avoidance of alcohol and other sedative agents that can worsen respiratory control, weight loss, improved sleep hygiene, regular exercise, and avoidance of sleep deprivation. The following discussion highlights the evidence-based treatment options for OSA. Use of complementary alternative therapies are beyond the scope of this review.

1.10.1 Surgery

The first line of treatment for pediatric OSA still continues to be adenotonsillectomy.

The landmark, randomized, controlled CHAT trial showed that children with OSA showed improvement in their condition with adenotonsillectomy, with reduced sleepiness and improved quality of life. Interestingly, there was no difference in attention and executive function between children with sleep apnea and those without [45]. Furthermore, almost half of the children who did not have surgery experienced an improvement on their own over a 7-month period [51]. The children who did undergo adenotonsillectomy, compared with watchful waiting, had improvements in parent-reported quality-of-life measures and OSA symptoms [52]. This has been confirmed in other studies. There is evidence of improvement in behavioral parameters, school performance, and quality of life improvement after treatment of OSA [53].

A recent meta-analysis on the role of tonsillectomy for obstructive sleep-disordered breathing involved 11 studies in children with follow-up of generally <1 year showed that there was an improvement in the AHI in children who received an adenotonsillectomy, in comparison with watchful waiting, which included three randomized, controlled trials [54, 55]. However, studies have demonstrated that the cure rate achieved with adenotonsillectomy is not nearly as substantial as was previously reported [56, 57]. A meta-analyses of these studies included predisposition toward asthma, obesity, age, and likely family history [58]. As the risks of surgery include postoperative bleeding and potentially death, there is a need for more thoughtful consideration about the role of surgery in treating the spectrum of sleep-disordered breathing and children (CHAT study) [59]. Recent approaches to address residual sleep apnea post adeno-tonsillectomy have used drug induced sleep endoscopy to target any surgical intervention. In a study of 20 pediatric patients, age 2-12 yrs, with residual OSA post-adenotonsillectomy, various surgeries have been performed using this type of endoscopy: total of 14 total tonsillectomies (70%), 7 with associated pharyngoplasties; 5 radiofrequency turbinate reductions (25%); 7 radio-frequency lingual tonsil reductions (35%); and 10 revision adenoidectomies (50%). No surgery-related complications were observed. The AHI scores at follow-up were significantly lower than AHI scores before surgery (1.895+/−1.11 vs 6.143+/−4.88; p<0.05) and, in 85% (n=17) of patients, the AHI was <3/hr. The outcome of drug-induced sleep endoscopy-directed surgery for persistent obstructive sleep apnea after adenotonsillar surgery [60] concludes that it is a useful and safe technique to decide a therapeutic strategy and to obtain good objective and subjective results regarding resolution of the syndrome. This suggests that targeted treatment approaches may be the optimal treatment method in the era of personalized medicine and children may need to undergo several interventions for potential cure.

Various surgical approaches are used in adults but are not indicated for pediatric OSA patients. One approach used in pediatrics and adults is lingual tonsillectomy. In a database review in 2013-2014, lingual tonsillectomies were performed in adults (mean age 36.5 yrs, 58% males) for obstructive sleep apnea as the most common indication for 58.7% of the 602 surgeries [61]. The resolution or efficacy was not reported. Upper airway surgery for OSA, across the continuum of the life-span, continues to evolve, ranging from uvulopalatopharyngoplasty to mandibular osteotomy with genioglossus advancement, mandibular distraction osteogenesis, sagittal split ramus osteotomy, hyoid myotomy, and bimaxillary advancement. Other techniques include osteogenic distraction radiofrequency ablation and possibly bariatric surgery for the treatment of OSA in obese patients.

1.10.2 Continuous Positive Airway Pressure Therapy

Continuous positive airway pressure (CPAP) therapy was invented over 25 years ago by Colin Sullivan. It consists of a portable device that provides a fan-generated continuous flow of air into the upper airway via a mask fitted over the nose and/or mouth, creating a pneumatic splint that prevents airway collapse associated with obstructive respiratory events. CPAP has been increasingly utilized in children. Its efficacy has been demonstrated, with improvements in sleep quality, daytime functioning, oxygenation, and ventilation [62–64]. Although the duration of use in adults is established, showing that longer use is associated with less sleepiness and improved respiratory outcomes, even use for as little as 2 h per night has correlated with improved behavioral outcomes in children. The biggest predictor of use in children is the maternal educational level, irrespective of the diagnosis, the age of the child, the severity of the sleep apnea, or developmental delay saem reference as above [63]. In addition, early and consistent use of CPAP predicts long-term use. Therefore, the first week of initiation of CPAP is most critical for troubleshooting to improve adherence and efficacy (Nixon et al). CPAP improves the AHI, decreases daytime sleepiness, and improves other parameters such as blood pressure, glycemic control, depression, and cognitive function [65]. The advances in the CPAP technology have exploded, resulting in better utilization, improved comfort, and a wide variety of interfaces, which can be individualized according to patient preference. The American Thoracic Society has recently published a patient education information series about positive airway pressure (PAP) therapy and tips for troubleshooting (PAP Therapy, American Thoracic Society, Patient Education, Information Series) [66]. Auto CPAP has also shown to be efficacious in children and adults [65, 67].

When CPAP was initially introduced, the titration was often performed within a laboratory setting. Advances in the technology have led to the development of autotitrating PAP devices with sophisticated wireless technology to not only treat but also monitor individuals on treatment.

Despite the efficacy of PAP treatment for children, there are some serious side effects to consider for long-term use of these devices. The interface of the PAP unit consists of a strap that goes behind the head of the child, and this create a continuous compressing force on the midface, resulting in stunting of the natural growth of the midface, which, in turn, has the potential to aggravate the structural component of OSAS. Unfortunately, this happens during the time at which the greatest cranial growth is occurring (at 4–6 years of age). By the age of 8 years, the skull has grown to over 90% of its adult size.

1.10.3 Medical Therapy

Medical therapy targeted two words each increasing inflammation of the airway, specifically decreasing the size of the tonsils and adenoids was first proposed over two decades ago. Several studies have independently demonstrated the role of inflammation-suppressing agents, such as inhaled corticosteroids and leukotriene receptor antagonists, in the treatment of OSA in children [68–70]. This is based on the premise that leukotrienes are inflammatory mediators and receptors for them have been found in the tonsils in children with OSA. At present, there is limited evidence to support wide use of this treatment, but there is emerging evidence to support its use [71–74]. In fact, there is a randomized, controlled trial in progress to address the role of intranasal steroids and leukotriene receptor antagonists in the treatment of OSA.

1.10.4 Mandibular Advancement Devices

Dental sleep medicine has expanded rapidly in the last two decades, and its role in the continuum of management of OSA is emerging. Some of the concepts are highlighted in detail in other chapters in this volume. The evidence in children suggests that mandibular advancement devices can help treat sleep apnea [50, 75]. Most of the evidence is based on studies performed by a selected group of researchers. Another study showed that use of a mandibular advancement device decreased NREM sleep instability in children with OSA [76]. The focus is changing from cosmetic dentistry to airway-based treatment in collaboration with pediatric otolaryngology and sleep medicine. Studies comparing appliances such as mandibular advancement devices and tongue retaining devices are generally less effective in reducing the AHI and the oxygen desaturation index than CPAP. However, symptom control is reported to be adequate in adults using oral appliances.

Despite the success of treatment of adult OSAS with oral appliances, these devices are not suitable for a growing individual; for that reason they are *contraindicated* for children. As the technology and science advance, there will likely be further delineation of individuals that may benefit from such devices for treating OSA.

1.10.5 Orthodontic/Dentofacial Orthopedics

The air that we breathe in can enter the body only through the nose and mouth. The nose is anatomically designed for breathing, and the mouth functions as a back-up airway entrance.

Any obstructions in this area will have an effect on the airflow to the body and consequently will increase resistance and create a partial or completely blockage. Orthodontic/dentofacial orthopedics has the greatest potential to improve OSAS; there are separate chapters dedicated to this treatment option elsewhere in this volume.

1.10.6 Other Therapies

Since it is clear that form and function both contribute to an airway that is affected by OSA, there is interest in exploring other surgical or medical targets for treatment. Myofunctional therapy involves training of the muscles to improve tongue tone and potentially decrease respiratory symptoms in children with OSA. In one study, 54 children (mean age 7 years) diagnosed with OSA were randomized to receive myofunctional therapy versus no treatment. The study showed that oropharyngeal exercises appear to effectively modify tongue tone, reduce OSA symptoms and oral breathing, and increase oxygen saturation, and may thus play a role in the treatment of OSA [77]. This therapy looks quite promising, but we are still uncertain of its role in all children. Villa et al. have substantial experience in treating these children by using dental and myofascial therapy.

1.11 Conclusions

Obstructive sleep apnea (OSA) is a highly prevalent medical disorder with significant associated sequelae in both children and adults. There are both genetic and environmental factors that can influence the onset and severity of OSA. It can occur throughout the life-span. The morbidity and mortality associated with OSA are significant, and it has widespread effects on cognitive performance, physical health, mood, and behavior. Therefore, screening for OSA should be integrated into health care visits. The treatment involves interdisciplinary cooperation to optimize the outcome and prevent sequelae, and ranges from medical therapy to orthodontics and surgery. Furthermore, the prevalence of this disorder in the context of other chronic disease is significant and has comorbidities that a comprehensive, multisystem and multimodal therapy will likely be required to substantially alleviate the burden of this disease.

References

1. Kryger M, Roth T, Dement W. Principles and practice of sleep medicine. 6th ed. Section 14. Philadelphia, PA: Elsvier; 2017.
2. Kushida CA. Obstructive sleep apnea: pathophysiology, comorbidities and consequences, vol. 1. Boca Raton, FL: CRC Press; 2007.
3. Marcus CL. Pathophysiology of childhood obstructive sleep apnea: current concepts. Respir Physiol. 2000;119(2–3):143–54. S0034568799001097 [pii].
4. Senaratna CV, Perret JL, Lodge CJ, Lowe AJ, Campbell BE, Matheson MC, Hamilton GS, Dharmage SC. Prevalence of obstructive sleep apnea in the general population: a systematic review. Sleep Med Rev. 2017;34:70–81.
5. American Academy of Sleep Medicine. The AASM manual for the scoring of sleep and associated events: rules, terminology and technical specifications (AASM Scoring Manual) version 2.4 2017.
6. Gottlieb DJ, Whitney CW, Bonekat WH, Iber C, James GD, Lebowitz M, et al. Relation of sleepiness to respiratory disturbance index: the Sleep Heart Health study. Am J Respir Crit Care Med. 1999;159(2):502–7.
7. Horne RS, Yang JS, Walter LM, Richardson HL, O'Driscoll DM, Foster AM, et al. Elevated blood pressure during sleep and wake in children with sleep-disordered breathing. Pediatrics. 2011;128(1):e85–92. https://doi.org/10.1542/peds.2010-3431.
8. AlGhanim N, Comondore VR, Fleetham J, Marra CA, Ayas NT. The economic impact of obstructive sleep apnea. Lung. 2008;186:7–12.
9. Ryan CM, Bradley TD. Pathogenesis of obstructive sleep apnea. J Appl Physiol. 2005;99:2440–50.
10. Wellman A, Genta PR, Owens RL, Edwards BA, Sands SA, Loring SH, White DP, Jackson AC, Pedersen OF, Butler JP. Test of the Starling resistor model in the human upper airway during sleep. J Appl Physiol (1985). 2014;117(12):1478–85. https://doi.org/10.1152/japplphysiol.00259.2014.

11. Wellman A, Genta P, et al. Test of the Starling resistor model in the human upper airway during sleep. J Appl Physiol (1985). 2014;117(12):1478–85.
12. Burgess K. New insights from the measurement of loop gain in obstructive sleep apnea. J Physiol. 2012;590(8):1781–2.
13. White LH, Motwani S, Kasai T, Yumino D, Amirthalingam V, Bradley TD. Effect of rostral fluid shift on pharyngeal resistance in men with and without obstructive sleep apnea. Respir Physiol Neurobiol. 2014;192:17–22.
14. Tapia IE, Bandla P, Traylor J, Karamessinis L, Huang J, Marcus CL. Upper airway sensory function in children with obstructive sleep apnea syndrome. Sleep. 2010;33(pg): 968–72.
15. Tapia IE, Kim JY, Cornaglia MA, Traylor J, et al. Upper airway vibration perception in school-aged children with obstructive sleep apnea. Sleep. 2016;39(9):1647–52.
16. Redline S, Tishler P. The genetics of sleep apnea. Sleep Med Rev. 2000;4(6):583–602.
17. Strohl KP, Redline S. Recognition of obstructive sleep apnea. Am J Respir Crit Care Med. 1996;154:279–89.
18. Taveira KVM, Kuntze MM, Berretta F, de Souza BDM, Godolfim LR, Demathe T, De Luca Canto G, Porporatti AL. Association between obstructive sleep apnea and alcohol, caffeine and tobacco: A meta-analysis. J Oral Rehabil. 2018;45(11):890–902.
19. Baker M, Scott B, Johnson RF, Mitchell RB. Predictors of obstructive sleep apnea severity in adolescents. JAMA Otolaryngol. 2017;143(5):494–9. https://doi.org/10.1001/jamaoto.2016.4130.
20. Glicksman A, Hadjiyannakis S, Barrowman N, Walker S, Hoey L, Katz SL. Body fat distribution ratios and obstructive sleep apnea severity in youth with obesity. J Clin Sleep Med. 2017;13(4):545–50. https://doi.org/10.5664/jcsm.6538.
21. Nelson HS. Advances in upper airway diseases and allergen immunotherapy. J Allergy Clin Immunol. 2006;117(5):1047–53.
22. Sakarya EU, Bayar Muluk N, Sakalar EG, Senturk M, Aricigil M, Bafaqeeh SA, et al. Use of intranasal corticosteroids in adenotonsillar hypertrophy. J Laryngol Otol. 2017;131(5):384–90. https://doi.org/10.1017/S0022215117000408.
23. Sullivan S, Li K, Guilleminault C. Nasal obstruction in children with sleep-disordered breathing. Ann Acad Med Singapore. 2008;37(8):645–8.
24. Cielo CM, Marcus CL. Obstructive sleep apnoea in children with craniofacial syndromes. Paediatr Respir Rev. 2015;16(3):189–96. https://doi.org/10.1016/j.prrv.2014.11.003.
25. Abdul Razak MR, Chirakalwasan N. Obstructive sleep apnea and asthma. Asian Pac J Allergy Immunol. 2016;34(4):265–71. https://doi.org/10.12932/AP0828.
26. Brockmann PE, Bertrand P, Castro-Rodriguez JA. Influence of asthma on sleep disordered breathing in children: a systematic review. Sleep Med Rev. 2014;18(5):393–7. https://doi.org/10.1016/j.smrv.2014.01.005.
27. Castro-Rodriguez JA, Brockmann PE, Marcus CL. Relation between asthma and sleep disordered breathing in children: is the association causal? Paediatr Respir Rev. 2017;22:72–5. S1526-0542(16)30084-7 [pii].
28. Ginis T, Akcan FA, Capanoglu M, Toyran M, Ersu R, Kocabas CN, et al. The frequency of sleep-disordered breathing in children with asthma and its effects on asthma control. J Asthma. 2017;54(4):403–10. https://doi.org/10.1080/02770903.2016.1220012.
29. Bhattacharjee R, Choi BH, Gozal D, Mokhlesi B. Association of adenotonsillectomy with asthma outcomes in children: a longitudinal database analysis. PLoS Med. 2014;11:e1001753.
30. Rodriguez JA, Brockmann P, Marcus CL. Relation between asthma and sleep disordered breathing in childrenL Is the association causal? Pediatr Respir Rev. 2017;(22):72–5.
31. Yerushalmy-Feler F, et al. Gluten-free diet may improve obstructive sleep apnea related symptoms in children with celiac disease. BMC Pediatr. 2018;18:35.
32. Gozal D. Sleep-disordered breathing and school performance in children. Pediatrics. 1998;102:61.
33. Gozal D, Pope DW Jr. Snoring during early childhood and academic performance at ages thirteen to fourteen years. Pediatrics. 2001;107(6):1394–9.

34. Chervin RD, Ruzicka DL, Giordani BJ, Weatherly RA, Dillon JE, Hodges EK, et al. Sleep-disordered breathing, behavior, and cognition in children before and after adenotonsillectomy. Pediatrics. 2006;117(4):e769–78. https://doi.org/10.1542/peds.2005-1837.
35. Beebe DW, Rausch J, Byars KC, Lanphear B, Yolton K. Persistent snoring in preschool children: predictors and behavioral and developmental correlates. Pediatrics. 2012;130(3):382–9. https://doi.org/10.1542/peds.2012-0045.
36. Young T, Palta M, Dempsey J, et al. The occurrence of sleep disordered breathing among middle-aged adults. N Engl J Med. 1993;328(17):1230–5.
37. West J, Luks AB. Respiratory physiology. The essentials. 10th ed. Philadelphia, PA: Wolters Kluwer. Lipponcott Williams, and Wilkins; 2016.
38. Fleck RJ, Shott SR, Mahmoud M, Ishman SL, Amin RS, Donnelly LF. Magnetic resonance imaging of obstructive sleep apnea in children. Pediatr Radiol. 2018;48(9):1223–33.
39. Ant A, Kemaloglu YK, Yilmaz M, Dilci A. Craniofacial deviations in the children with nasal obstruction. J Craniofac Surg. 2017;28(3):625–8. https://doi.org/10.1097/SCS.0000000000003409.
40. Kapur VK, et al. Clinical practice guideline for diagnostic testing for adult obstructive sleep apnea: An American academy of sleep medicine clinical practice guideline. J Clin Sleep Med. 2017;13(3):479–504.
41. Rosen IM, Kirsch DB, Chervin RD, Carden KA, Ramar K, Aurora RN, Kristo DA, Malhotra RK, Martin JL, Olson EJ, Rosen CL, Rowley JA. Clinical use of a home sleep apnea test: An American academy of sleep medicine position statement. J Clin Sleep Med. 2017;13(10):1205–7.
42. Alvarez D, Alonso-Alvarez ML, Gutierrez-Tobal GC, Crespo A, Kheirandish-Gozal L, Hornero R, et al. Automated screening of children with obstructive sleep apnea using nocturnal oximetry: an alternative to respiratory polygraphy in unattended settings. J Clin Sleep Med. 2017;13(5):693–702. https://doi.org/10.5664/jcsm.6586.
43. Hornero R, Kheirandish-Gozal L, Gutierrez-Tobal GC, Philby MF, Alonso-Alvarez ML, Alvarez D, et al. Nocturnal oximetry-based evaluation of habitually snoring children. Am J Respir Crit Care Med. 2017;196:1591. https://doi.org/10.1164/rccm.201705-0930OC.
44. Rosen CL, Wang R, Taylor HG, Marcus CL, Katz ES, Paruthi S, et al. Utility of symptoms to predict treatment outcomes in obstructive sleep apnea syndrome. Pediatrics. 2015;135(3):e662–71. https://doi.org/10.1542/peds.2014-3099.
45. Mitchell RB, Garetz S, Moore RH, Rosen CL, Marcus CL, Katz ES, et al. The use of clinical parameters to predict obstructive sleep apnea syndrome severity in children: the Childhood Adenotonsillectomy (CHAT) study randomized clinical trial. JAMA Otolaryngol. 2015;141(2):130–6. https://doi.org/10.1001/jamaoto.2014.3049.
46. Konstantinopoulou S, Gallagher P, Elden L, Garetz SL, Mitchell RB, Redline S, et al. Complications of adenotonsillectomy for obstructive sleep apnea in school-aged children. Int J Pediatr Otorhinolaryngol. 2015;79(2):240–5. https://doi.org/10.1016/j.ijporl.2014.12.018.
47. Alsufyani N, Isaac A, Witmans M, Major P, El-Hakim H. Predictors of failure of DISE-directed adenotonsillectomy in children with sleep disordered breathing. J Otolaryngol Head Neck Surg. 2017;46(1):37. https://doi.org/10.1186/s40463-017-0213-3.
48. Brown KA, Morin I, Hickey C, Manoukian JJ, Nixon GM, Brouillette RT. Urgent adenotonsillectomy: an analysis of risk factors associated with postoperative respiratory morbidity. Anesthesiology. 2003;99(3):586–95.
49. Villa MP, Bernkopf E, Pagani J, Broia V, Montesano M, Ronchetti R. Randomized controlled study of an oral jaw-positioning appliance for the treatment of obstructive sleep apnea in children with malocclusion. Am J Respir Crit Care Med. 2002;165(1):123–7.
50. Villa MP, Malagola C, Pagani J, Montesano M, Rizzoli A, Guilleminault C, et al. Rapid maxillary expansion in children with obstructive sleep apnea syndrome: 12-month follow-up. Sleep Med. 2007;8(2):128–34.
51. Chervin RD, Ellenberg SS, Hou X, Marcus CL, Garetz SL, Katz ES, et al. Prognosis for spontaneous resolution of OSA in children. Chest. 2015;148(5):1204–13. S0012-3692(15)50231-6 [pii].

52. Garetz SL, Mitchell RB, Parker PD, Moore RH, Rosen CL, Giordani B, et al. Quality of life and obstructive sleep apnea symptoms after pediatric adenotonsillectomy. Pediatrics. 2015;135(2):e477–86. https://doi.org/10.1542/peds.2014-0620.
53. Mitchell RB, Kelly J. Behavior, neurocognition and qualityof-life in children with sleep-disordered breathing. Int J Pediatr Otorhinolaryngol. 2006;70:395–406.
54. Marcus CL. Tonsillectomy for short-term benefit in obstructive sleep-disordered breathing. J Pediatr. 2017;186:209–12. S0022-3476(17)30502-4 [pii].
55. Chinnadurai S, Jordan AK, Sathe NA, Fonnesbeck C, McPheeters ML, Francis DO. Tonsillectomy for obstructive sleep-disordered breathing: a meta-analysis. Pediatrics. 2017;139(2):e20163491. https://doi.org/10.1542/peds.2016-3491.
56. Mitchell RB, Archer SM, Ishman SL, Rosenfeld RM, Coles S, Finestone SA, Friedman NR, Giordano T, Hildrew DM, Kim TW, Lloyd RM, Parikh SR, Shulman ST, Walner DL, Walsh SA, Nnacheta LC. Clinical practice guideline: tonsillectomy in children (update). Otolaryngol Head Neck Surg. 2019 Feb;160(1_suppl):S1–S42.
57. Tauman R, Gulliver TE, Krishna J, Montgomery-Downs HE, O'Brien LM, Ivanenko A, et al. Persistence of obstructive sleep apnea syndrome in children after adenotonsillectomy. J Pediatr. 2006;149(6):803–8.
58. Bhattacharjee R, Kheirandish-Gozal L, Spruyt K, Mitchell RB, Promchiarak J, Simakajornboon N, et al. Adenotonsillectomy outcomes in treatment of obstructive sleep apnea in children: a multicenter retrospective study. Am J Respir Crit Care Med. 2010;182(5):676–83.
59. Marcus C, Moore R, Rosen C, et al. A randomized Trial of adenotonsillectomy for Childhood Sleep Apnea Published in final edited form as. N Engl J Med. 2013;368(25):2366–76. Published online 2013 May 21.
60. Esteller E, Villatoro JC, Aguero A, Matino E, Lopez R, Aristimuno A, Nunez V, Diaz-Herrera MA. Outcome of drug-induced sleep endoscopy-directed surgery for persistent obstructive sleep apnea after adenotonsillar surgery. Int J Pediatr Otorhinolaryngol. 2019;120:118–22.
61. Merna C, Lin HW, Bhattacharyya N. Clinical characteristics, complications, and reasons for readmission following lingual tonsillectomy. Otolaryngol Head Neck Surg. 2019;160(4): 619–21. https://doi.org/10.1177/0194599819827820.
62. Sawyer AM, Gooneratne NS, Marcus CL, Ofer D, Richards KC, Weaver TE. A systematic review of CPAP adherence across age groups: clinical and empiric insights for developing CPAP adherence interventions. Sleep Med Rev. 2011;15(6):343–56.
63. Marcus CL, Radcliffe J, Konstantinopoulou S, Beck SE, Cornaglia MA, Traylor J, DiFeo N, Karamessinis LR, Gallagher PR, Meltzer LJ. Effects of positive airway pressure therapy on neurobehavioral outcomes in children with obstructive sleep apnea. Am J Respir Crit Care Med. 2012;185(9):998–1003. https://doi.org/10.1164/rccm.201112-2167OC.
64. Horne RSC. Investing in the future: the benefits of continuous positive airway pressure for childhood obstructive sleep apnea. Am J Respir Crit Care Med. 2012;185(9):908–10. https://doi.org/10.1164/rccm.201202-0296ED.
65. Patil SP, Ayappa IA, Caples SM, Kimoff RJ, Patel SR, Harrod CG. Treatment of adult obstructive sleep apnea with positive airway pressure: an American academy of sleep medicine clinical practice guideline. J Clin Sleep Med. 2019;15(2):335–43.
66. American Thoracic Society. PAP therapy—tips for troubleshooting to address problems with use. Patient Education Information Series. https://www.thoracic.org/patients/patient-resources/resources/paptroubleshooting.pdf. Accessed Sep 2016.
67. Mihai R, Vandeleur M, Pecoraro S, Davey MJ, Nixon GM. Autotitrating CPAP as a Tool for CPAP Initiation for Children. J Clin Sleep Med. 2017;13(5):713–9.
68. de Benedictis FM, Bush A. Corticosteroids in respiratory diseases in children. Am J Respir Crit Care Med. 2012;185:12.
69. Goldbart AD, Goldman JL, Veling MC, Gozal D. Leukotriene modifier therapy for mild sleep-disordered breathing in children. Am J Respir Crit Care Med. 2005;172(3):364–70.
70. Kheirandish-Gozal L, Serpero LD, Dayyat E, Kim J, Goldman JL, Snow A, et al. Corticosteroids suppress in vitro tonsillar proliferation in children with obstructive sleep apnoea. Eur Respir J. 2009;33(5):1077–84.

71. Dayyat E, Serpero LD, Kheirandish-Gozal L, Goldman JL, Snow A, Bhattacharjee R, et al. Leukotriene pathways and in vitro adenotonsillar cell proliferation in children with obstructive sleep apnea. Chest. 2009;135(5):1142–9.
72. Canadian Agency for Drugs and Technologies in Health [CADTH]. Montelukast for sleep apnea: a review of the clinical effectiveness, cost effectiveness, and guidelines. Ottawa, ON: CADTH; 2014.
73. Satdhabudha A, Sritipsukho P, Manochantr S, Chanvimalueng W, Chaumrattanakul U, Chaumphol P. Urine cysteinyl leukotriene levels in children with sleep disordered breathing before and after adenotonsillectomy. Int J Pediatr Otorhinolaryngol. 2017;94:112–6. S0165-5876(17)30036-8 [pii].
74. Sunkonkit K, Sritippayawan S, Veeravikrom M, Deerojanawong J, Prapphal N. Urinary cysteinyl leukotriene E4 level and therapeutic response to montelukast in children with mild obstructive sleep apnea. Asian Pac J Allergy Immunol. 2017;35:233. https://doi.org/10.12932/AP0879.
75. Boudewyns A, Abel F, Alexopoulos E, Evangelisti M, Kaditis A, Miano S, et al. Adenotonsillectomy to treat obstructive sleep apnea: is it enough? Pediatr Pulmonol. 2017;52(5):699–709. https://doi.org/10.1002/ppul.23641.
76. Miano S, Rizzoli A, Evangelisti M, Bruni O, Ferri R, Pagani J, et al. NREM sleep instability changes following rapid maxillary expansion in children with obstructive apnea sleep syndrome. Sleep Med. 2009;10(4):471–8.
77. Villa MP, Evangelisti M, Martella S, Barreto M, Del Pozzo M. Can myofunctional therapy increase tongue tone and reduce symptoms in children with sleep-disordered breathing? Sleep Breath. 2017;21:1025. https://doi.org/10.1007/s11325-017-1489-2.

Signs and Symptoms of Non-restorative Sleep

2

Osman S. Ipsiroglu

2.1 Overview and Concepts: Sleep/Wake Behaviours Assessments in Clinical Practice of Non-sleep Experts

2.1.1 Introduction

Through my daily clinical work in developmental paediatrics and child and adolescent psychiatry, I have seen an increasing number of children and youth with neurodevelopmental and/or neuropsychiatric conditions, who suffer from undiagnosed and/or untreated sleep problems. I came to the realization that the lack of attention given to these problems by medical care providers came from the scarcity of *explanatory models* for reported symptoms. All patients had received various developmental paediatrics and mental health diagnoses, based on their daytime presentations (e.g. attention deficit hyperactivity disorder, ADHD; autism spectrum disorder, autism). However, the possible effect that chronic sleep deprivation had on daytime symptoms was either *recognized* but *not investigated further* or *remained unrecognized* and was therefore *taken as given* or even considered to be *part of the condition*.

Inspired by *Charles Dickens*, I decided to approach clinical encounters from a medical anthropology and educational psychology viewpoint. Applying the concepts of *ethnography* and *ecology* helped me to discover the inadequacies of the current clinical explanatory models, which overlooked children's sleep problems [1]. In clinical practice, *ethnography* refers to neutral (unconfounded or unbiased) exploration of a patient [2–4] and *ecology* recognizes the importance of respecting

O. S. Ipsiroglu (✉)
Department of Paediatrics, Faculty of Medicine, University of British Columbia, Vancouver, BC, Canada

H-Behaviours Research Lab [Previously Sleep/Wake-Behaviour Research Lab], BC Children's Hospital Research Institute, University of British Columbia, Vancouver, BC, Canada
e-mail: oipsiroglu@bcchr.ca

© Springer Nature Switzerland AG 2019
E. Liem (ed.), *Sleep Disorders in Pediatric Dentistry*,
https://doi.org/10.1007/978-3-030-13269-9_2

the complex interconnections in the lives of patients [5–8]. Integrating ethnography and ecology during clinical encounters automatically leads to bidirectional communication or explorative interviewing. Explorative interviewing exceeds unidirectional communication and can help clinicians overcome misunderstandings with patients and develop a shared language among all involved parties. This article gives an overview of how, during clinical encounters, *the description of behaviours and clinical features* as *clinical best practice* can change our understanding of sleep problems in children with neurodevelopmental and/or neuropsychiatric conditions.

2.1.2 Preface: A Plea for Explorative Interviewing

This chapter was written for practitioners with backgrounds in medicine, dentistry, or rehabilitation and professionals who encounter orofacial morphology or functioning during their work in orthodontics, oral surgery, sleep medicine, physiotherapy, physical medicine, paediatric dentistry, otolaryngology, occupational therapy, speech-language pathology, myofunctional therapy, dental hygiene, and lactation consulting. Independent of background, training, and discipline, the goal of this chapter is to convey to readers the importance of developing a shared language and bidirectional communication with patients, to increase mutual understanding of the most common sleep problems and find effective therapeutic solutions. It is devoted to Charles Dickens, the well-known British novelist, who was able to describe the entire dimension of sleep-disordered breathing (SDB) in his book, *The Pickwick Papers* (serialized in 1836 and published in book format in 1837, [9]). He accomplished this task 160 years before the American Academy of Sleep Medicine released their consensus statement about sleep-disordered breathing [10, 11]. *How could a writer, who had never studied medicine, describe the entire spectrum of SDB so accurately almost 200 years before contemporary scientists?* Dickens' detailed and empathetic case report of SDB is based on his objective, curiosity-driven, and neutral observational skills and should encourage us to review clinical challenges similarly without missing the big picture. Thus, this chapter addresses the shortfalls of academic sleep lab-based research and offers clinical practitioners an *explorative best practice* approach.

2.2 Sleep Problems in Children with Neurodevelopmental and/or Neuropsychiatric Conditions: *Adoption of an Orphan into Medical Concepts or Why We Do Need an Explorational Interviewing Concept?*

2.2.1 Aetiological and Neurophysiological Aspects

2.2.1.1 Sleep
Sleep is a neurologic, restorative function that is essential for childhood development, physical health, cognitive function, and psycho-mental well-being [12]. Consequently, sleep problems should be of particular concern in children with neurodevelopmental and/or neuropsychiatric conditions. In the first comprehensive

review of sleep habits of children with neurodevelopmental and/or neuropsychiatric conditions affecting sleep and sleep/wake behaviours, Jan et al. [13] estimated a 75–80% prevalence rate of chronic sleep problems for these children, in contrast to 30–35% prevalence in otherwise healthy children [13]. A majority of these sleep problems manifest themselves as insomnia, difficulties in falling asleep and maintaining sleep, resulting in chronic sleep deprivation [14–17].

2.2.1.2 Sleep Deprivation

Sleep deprivation in children generally manifests itself as daytime inattention, hyperactivity, and mood disturbances [18, 19]; this is also the case in patients with neurodevelopmental and/or neuropsychiatric conditions [13]. However, among these children, sleep problems are only one of many different types of medical problems and, as a result, often go undiagnosed and untreated [15]. Moreover, the causal role of sleep problems in children's behaviours and in their entire clinical picture may be underestimated or remain unrecognized [20].

2.2.1.3 Spectrum of Sleep Disorders

Most sleep problems encountered in children with neurodevelopmental and/or neuropsychiatric conditions are due to a myriad of conditions affecting multiple organ systems and functions, which are essential prerequisites for a normal sleep. Conditions include craniofacial malformations (e.g. cleft palate syndromes, high-arched palate), neuromuscular disorders (e.g. Duchenne-Becker muscular dystrophy), rare biochemical disorders (e.g. mucopolysaccharidoses), obesity, Down syndrome, and the neurologic disorder, Willis-Ekbom disease/restless legs syndrome (WED/RLS). The underlying pathophysiology includes upper airway obstructions, muscle weakness impacting respiratory drive, reduced secretion of sleep-related hormones (mainly melatonin) and neurotransmitters (e.g. dopaminergic substances), and sensorimotor symptoms. Further, epilepsy (e.g. manifesting as seizures during the night), discomfort or pain, hunger or gastrointestinal tract irritation (e.g. through nocturnal gastrostomy tube feeding), and side effects of pharmacological treatments are additional causes of sleep problems in children with neurodevelopmental and/or neuropsychiatric conditions. Psychological trauma, mental health disorders (e.g. ADHD), but also autism spectrum disorders, prenatal alcohol exposure, congenital or acquired brain injuries, and various forms of cerebral palsy are almost invariably associated with sleep problems. Pathophysiological targets for specific treatments of sleep problems are widely unknown; therefore, therapies mainly focus on interventions targeting daytime symptoms.

2.2.1.4 Sleep-Disordered Breathing

Research on sleep-disordered breathing has mainly been conducted in the domain of lab-based research for the last 35 years. It focused initially on infants with periodic breathing, as well as on central and obstructive apnoea. The focus then shifted to the broader spectrum of sleep-disordered breathing and included hypopnea, upper airway restrictions, and flow limitations. Recently, it has been recognized that in addition to lack of oxygen, desaturation and limb movement-associated arousals can result in a fragmentation of sleep and are one of the main causes of non-restorative disturbed sleep.

2.2.1.5 Insomnia in Children

Insomnia in children has been mainly conceptualized as a behavioural problem as almost all children, due to secondary 'learned behaviours', caused some parental insomnia [21]. Successful analysis of potential causes for behavioural insomnia led paediatricians, psychologists, and researchers to focus on sleep hygiene measures, which were investigated and analysed from various aspects [12]. The reviews of sleep hygiene/health measures of children with neurodevelopmental and/or neuropsychiatric conditions, which framed the clinical practice and research at our Sleep/Wake Behaviour Clinic of the last decade, impressively demonstrated the limitations in our understanding and the need for more phenomenological research into the causes of insomnia in children [13, 14, 22].

2.2.1.6 Willis-Ekbom Disease/Restless Legs Syndrome (WED/RLS)

Recently, there has been renewed interest among sleep researchers in WED/RLS symptoms in children and adolescents [23]. The clinical picture of WED/RLS is well known in adults and was first described by Sir Thomas Willis in 1672 [24]. Most adults suffering from WED/RLS describe that they first experienced symptoms at a very young age. WED/RLS may cause delayed sleep onset in children with neurodevelopmental and/or neuropsychiatric conditions and can contribute significantly to childhood insomnia. Also, the discomfort of suppressing the urge to move most likely delays pineal melatonin production and secretion. The delayed recognition of WED/RLS as a main cause of insomnia is a puzzling observation, as WED/RLS typically accompanies sensory processing abnormalities, and many children with neurodevelopmental and/or neuropsychiatric conditions experience major sensory processing difficulties already at a very young age [25].

2.2.2 Sleep and Neurodevelopmental and/or Neuropsychiatric Conditions

Sleep is an integral component of cerebral function and a prerequisite for the development of cognitive, emotional, and behavioural skills. The negative impact of sleep problems on child development has been well documented [26, 27]. Transient sleep problems are highly prevalent across all ages and cause major problems [28]; chronic sleep problems have devastating consequences as they adversely affect cognition, emotion, and behaviours [29, 30]. However, the degree to which early-onset and chronic sleep problems in children with underlying developmental conditions can contribute to (a) aggravation of developmental delay or intellectual disability and (b) mental health disorders or (c) trigger misdiagnosis and overmedication has not been investigated. Given the fact that up to 20% of children and adolescents live with chronic physical, neurodevelopmental and/or neuropsy-chiatric, and behavioural or emotional conditions [31], and up to 80% of these children suffer from chronic sleep problems [13, 29, 32], we consider sleep as a main factor affecting well-being and quality of life of affected children and their families/caregivers.

2.3   The Sleep/Wake Behaviours Assessment

2.3.1   A Face-to-Face History Taking

The clinical and narrative sleep/wake behaviours history taking is conducted as a semi-structured explorative face-to-face interview (without a desk obstructing the view to the patient and/or accompanying parents). For facilitating visualization of experienced challenges, the patient/parents are encouraged to narrate the sleep- and wake-related behaviours of their child in their own words and in the context of everyday routines with descriptions [1, 33]. Special emphasis is given to transitioning behaviours during day-, bed-, and night-time, as well as daytime resting activities. BEARS domains (bedtime, excessive daytime sleepiness, awakenings, regularity/routines, and snoring) [34] are explored with standard questions (such as how often? and since when?) with an emphasis on urge-to-move patterns in the first four domains. To further support the clinical assessment and develop a more comprehensive clinical picture, some adaptations were made to the BEARS [35] (Table 2.1). Snoring was changed to sleep-disordered breathing, and facial cues that might signify breathing difficulties are captured. In positive cases, symptoms are further investigated with the Sleep Disturbance Scale for Children (SDSC) [37] and/or the pediatric sleep questionnaire (PSQ) [38]. Additional areas for developing a holistic understanding included medical and functional diagnoses of co-morbidities, ongoing therapies, medications and medication effects (psychotropic medications in particular), and scales for subjective assessment of how symptoms impact the well-being of the child and caregivers. *The extended sleep/wake behaviours family history* includes questions addressing familial sleep disturbances associated with non-restorative sleep (e.g. snoring, dry mouth, sweating, restlessness during sleep) and WED/RLS-related symptoms (e.g. behaviours during TV watching as an example for restful activity in the evening, quality of sleep, e.g. deep or light sleeper, restful or restless sleeper, and awakening behaviours), as well as history of familial iron deficiency. This extended history captures the dimensions of non-restorative sleep with a focus on sleep-disordered breathing, insomnia, and the family sleep habits, thus supporting the development of a shared language (Table 2.1).

2.3.2   Standardized Description of (Behavioural) Observations and Functioning

2.3.2.1 Facial Anatomical Features

Independent of craniofacial conditions/malformations (e.g. cleft palate, Apert syndrome) and space assessment via the Mallampati score, mandibular positioning (retrognathia, overflow), maxillary hypoplasia, high-arched palate and teeth positioning, and functional observations such as mouth/nose breathing and oromotor hypotonia should be reviewed and investigated. *The suggested clinical immobilization test (SCIT)* allows for standardized observations of behaviours and movements with/without an electromyography (EMG). The SCIT is administered to both the child and the parent(s) (see Fig. 2.1a); in cases where the SCIT cannot be

Table 2.1 Clinical sleep/wake history taking

Clinical assessment categories	Descriptions
B	Bedtime situations which facilitate the patient's ability to fall asleep 1. For example, during passive transfers are further explored (i.e. "how long does it take him/her to fall asleep in the stroller or during a car ride?") 2. Movement patterns, including gestalt of these movement patterns prior to falling asleep, immediately after falling asleep, and during resting situations when awake (i.e. "how still can he/she be in the car seat, can you describe his/her movement patterns?"), are further explored
E	Excessive daytime sleepiness was altered to excessive daytime behaviours, as hyperactive-like behaviours are explored ex aequo, also perceptions about stressful daytime situations in accounts that relate to the well-being of the child (and themselves)
A	Awakenings, parasomnias, and rhythmic movement disorders are explored. Parents are encouraged to elaborate about their perceptions of stressful night-time situations and restorative/non-restorative sleep perception in accounts that relate to the well-being of the child (and themselves)
R	Routines and regularity (e.g. hours of sleep) are asked with special focus on transitioning situations (i.e. from movement to rest and vice versa, e.g. at school or during dinner), in addition to sleep health measures
S	Snoring was changed to sleep-disordered breathing, and signs of sleep-disordered breathing, such as open-mouth posture, signs of non-restorative sleep (restless/sweating), and problems in getting up in the morning were screened
Non-restorative sleep	Waking up not refreshed despite having enough hours of sleep
Well-being (quality of life)	Ranking of current well-being and well-being if sleep problems improved, on a scale from 0 (lowest) to 10 (highest) for patient and parent/caregiver(s)

As a qualitative exploratory interviewing approach of best/worst sleep/wake situations, we use the modified mnemonic (Vancouver Polar BEARS) [35], which also includes questions about (1) family ecology [6, 7, 36], e.g. "can you give some descriptions related to the child's strengths and problem behaviour and how these affect the child, you, and your family?" [1]; (2) child development, e.g. describing his/her development and behaviour and describing sleep patterns and any breathing or sensory problems; (3) any sleep/wake behaviours treatments, e.g. what efforts have been made to improve sleep?; and (4) the impact of sleep problem on the family, e.g. how did your child's sleep problem impact your life/the life of your family and the life of the child? From "De-medicalizing sleep: sleep assessment tools in the community setting for clients (patients) with FASD & prenatal substance exposure," by O. S. Ipsiroglu, N. Carey, J. Collet, D. Fast, J. Garden, J. E. Jan., … M. Witmans, 2012, *National Organisation for Fetal Alcohol Syndrome – UK (NOFAS-UK): Fetal Alcohol Forum*. Copyright 2012 by NOFAS-UK

administered (e.g. due to lack of comprehension, behavioural compliance, or motor ability), observations of the child (with shoes and socks removed) while moving around, coming to rest, and starting movements again in the examination room can be used instead ([25]; informal SCIT; see Fig. 2.1b). Explaining the observations from the SCIT to the parents usually triggers additional narratives of related information about similar situations at home.

a

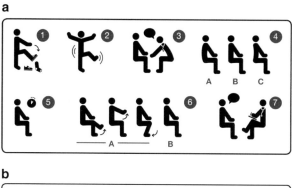

b

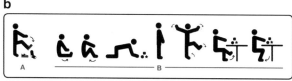

Fig. 2.1 (**a**) Formal SCIT procedure. Clinician asks the participant to (1) remove their socks/
shoes; (2) stand up, stretch, and shake out; and (3) sit down in a heightwise appropriately sized
chair. Clinician interacts with participant until he/she feels relaxed (e.g. by telling a joke or lightly
shaking the participant's knee(s): relaxation might trigger sensations, an urge to move, and/or
involuntary H-movements). (4) Pre-SCIT: clinician observes participant's sitting position
("gestalt of posture"), (A) relaxed, (B) inconclusive, and (C) tense. (5) SCIT: clinician asks
participant to sit in a relaxed way for up to a maximum of 5 min with their feet flat on the floor
and observes the participant. The time can be shortened if the participant can describe the
sensations or the urge to move; usually there are short movements, and after discussing them the
entire procedure should be repeated starting from 2 (getting up and shaking out). (6) Post-SCIT:
clinician indicates that the test is over and observes any compensatory movement patterns (to get
rid of discomfort) and/or (in)voluntary movements the participant has after the test, (A) significant
movement patterns and (B) minimal to no movement patterns. (7) Clinician explores again any
sensations and movement patterns the participant has felt during the SCIT and/or post-SCIT. From
"Video Recordings of Naturalistic Observations: Pattern Recognition of Disruptive Behaviours in
People with Mental Health or Neurodevelopmental Conditions," by O. S. Ipsiroglu, G. Kloesch,
N. Beyzaei, S. McCabe, M. Berger, H. J. Kuhle, … H. Garn, 2017, Brücken bauen:
Kinderschlafmedizin verbindet - Aktuelle Kinderschlafmedizin 2017 [Building Bridges:
Combining Pediatric Sleep Medicine - Current Pediatric Sleep Medicine 2017] (pp. 54–76).
Copyright 2017 by Kleanthes Verlag für Medizin und Prävention. Reprinted with permission. (**b**)
Informal SCIT procedure. In cases where the full SCIT cannot be administered (e.g. due to lack
of comprehension, behavioural compliance, or motor ability), (A) observations of the child (with
shoes and socks removed) while (B) moving around, coming to rest, and starting movements
again in the examination room should be used instead. From "Video Recordings of Naturalistic
Observations: Pattern Recognition of Disruptive Behaviours in People with Mental Health or
Neurodevelopmental Conditions," by O. S. Ipsiroglu, G. Kloesch, N. Beyzaei, S. McCabe,
M. Berger, H. J. Kuhle, … H. Garn, 2017, Brücken bauen: Kinderschlafmedizin verbindet -
Aktuelle Kinderschlafmedizin 2017 [Building Bridges: Combining Pediatric Sleep Medicine -
Current Pediatric Sleep Medicine 2017] (pp. 54–76). Copyright 2017 by Kleanthes Verlag für
Medizin und Prävention. Reprinted with permission

2.3.2.2 Exploration of Sensory Processing Abnormalities (SPAs)

During the assessment (usually following the SCIT), parents are asked to identify (1) if their child had experienced any SPAs ("Does your child have any sensory processing challenges?" and "Have sensory processing challenges been mentioned by any health care professionals?"). (a) If yes, the types of experienced SPAs were further explored with narratives provided by the parent(s) (e.g. "He/she must wear clothes with the labels removed".). The pain threshold of the child and affected family members is further explored in each case. (b) If no, sensory challenges are further explored with specific questions about the inability to integrate and respond to sensory stimuli appropriately ("Does your child show any responses to touch or auditory stimuli which you consider different from your own responses or that of other children or his/her peers?"). Parents are also asked to identify (2) whether a formal sensory assessment had been conducted by an occupational therapist trained in assessing sensory problems.

2.3.3 Quality Control

2.3.3.1 Sleep/Wake Behaviours Reports

The end product of the assessment is a sleep/wake behaviours report, including (1) a detailed description and summary of sleep/wake behaviours (including excerpts of original quotations by patients/parents); (2) interpretations for healthcare providers, incorporating the parents' narrative in plain language, i.e. avoiding medical terminology; (3) and recommendations for parents, and community-based support teams (if involved). We used inclusive language at a grade-five reading level [1, 33]. Parents were asked to review and edit the reports in collaboration with the healthcare professionals involved in the assessment [39, 40]. Complex cases were followed up and discussed with involved community-based paediatricians and therapy teams.

> *Implications for Best Practice in the Community: Explorative interviewing in clinical encounters supports the creation of bidirectional communication and strengthens therapeutic relationships. It is applied in various ways by all professionals; there are subgroups of professionals, who apply it due to the nature of their service (e.g. occupational therapists), whereas some subspecialists might not have the time for bidirectional communication (e.g. in the emergency room during triage). In children with neurodevelopmental and/or neuropsychiatric conditions, sleep/wake behaviours assessments have to be conducted via explorative interviewing.*

2.3.4 "What Are the Consequences of Unrecognized Sleep Problems?"

Undiagnosed chronic sleep problems pave the way for overmedication and polypharmacy in adolescents with FASDs, autism, and Down syndrome.

Our *initial observation* was that none of these children and adolescents had been assessed systematically with a relevant open-ended screening questionnaire [34] or a more formal diagnostic questionnaire [38, 41, 42] prior to the prescription of sleep medication and other symptomatic strategies for intractable chronic insomnia. Eventually, after the initial medication proved ineffective in treating the sleep problems, patients were then referred to our clinic for formal systematic assessments [1].

The *second core observation* was prescription of multiple, off-label, and concurrent pharmaceutical medications [43]. We performed in-depth analysis of the challenging/disruptive sleep and wake behaviours and medication history of 17 adolescent patients with a pharmacotherapy timeline. We captured (1) the medications and order of prescriptions and (2) the age at the time of first prescription. All patients presented with intractable chronic insomnia and fulfilled the diagnostic criteria for familial WED/RLS. Eleven of 17 had additional clinical signs of SDB, and 14/17 showed excessive daytime behaviours (sleepiness and/or hyperactive-like behaviours to fight fatigue/sleepiness). The medication analysis revealed two prescription strategies: (a) targeting sleep problems with melatonin, second-generation antipsychotics, and/or a combination of both (10/17) and (b) targeting hyperactive-like daytime behaviours with a psychostimulant (7/10). In addition, many medications were prescribed in combination and at alarmingly young ages [43]. One 4.5-year-old patient with an FASD was prescribed a psychostimulant, and another patient with autism was prescribed a second-generation antipsychotic at 2.5 years of age.

Our *third observation* was that the prescription strategies for children with autism under 6 years started to change over the last decade: recently, children with autism below the age of 6 are less medicated [44]. Our understanding is that the focus on behavioural therapeutic interventions has highlighted sleep problems among children with autism [15], and recently a more thoughtful prescription pattern has emerged. This includes a review of the need for iron supplementation [45] or the need to address sensory processing abnormalities [46].

Implications for Best Practice in the Community: Vulnerable patient groups, like children and adolescents with neurodevelopmental and/or neuropsychiatric conditions, are at particular risk for iatrogenic harm due to gaps in our clinical understanding and lack of time for in-depth investigations. New clinical research priorities include examining the association between behavioural or neurologic adverse drug reactions to psychostimulants and antipsychotics and challenging/disruptive sleep and wake behaviours in patients with WED/RLS, whose insomnia and/or non-restorative sleep was triggered by medications.

2.4   Results

2.4.1   Non-restorative Sleep: Diagnostic Versus Explorational History Taking

The main reason why professionals who practise in community settings need a new perspective on non-restorative sleep in children (and most probably in geriatric patients) is because current diagnostic criteria for SDB and WED/RLS are based on descriptions by parents/caregivers or self-description. While in SDB the gold standard for diagnosis is polysomnography (PSG) [47], there is no device-based gold standard for the diagnosis of WED/RLS [48]. Periodic limb movements (PLMs) in sleep can support the diagnosis of WED/RLS [23], but access to polysomnography is limited in many geographical regions around the world (including Canada). *How can we optimize our clinical understanding and try to describe the relationship between non-restorative sleep and excessive daytime behaviours better?*

The proposed concept of structured observations in the context of explorational history taking can be applied during an office visit and provides information on factors that put a patient at high risk for SDB and/or WED/RLS. Why is this necessary?

1. Because of *Communication Barriers*. The complex biographies of patients contribute to "communication barriers". These barriers are often related to the common medical practice of diagnostic history taking, utilizing checklists, leading to unidirectional communication due to time constraints [49].
2. Because *Conventional Daytime-Focused Mainstream Views* need to be challenged. Clinical explorational history taking and reviews of patients' records verified that symptoms were identified, but not attributed to possible sleep problems as an aggravating factor. All diagnoses were complicated by multiple co-morbidities [1, 25]. Most striking was that children with a prenatal alcohol exposure [35] and an autism diagnosis beyond the age of 6 [44], respectively, had been medicated for sleep problems (including chloral hydrate and atypical antipsychotics) without a systematic reproducible assessment. The in-depth clinical investigations revealed that many of these children had behaviours not previously reported in their histories, including disordered breathing and probable familial WED/RLS. These conditions, which had not been investigated previously, may have contributed to a significant degree to the FASD- or autism-related multiple co-morbidities [50]. In other words, the current diagnostic history taking of professionals did not recognize sleep problems as a distinct category for clinical investigation and diagnosis that encompassed both daytime and night-time well-being and behaviour. In summary, clinical investigations revealed that the provision of a categorical diagnosis of prenatal alcohol exposure and/or autism obscured the need for full functional assessment and intervention [1, 44].
3. Because of *Missing Knowledge*. The examination of the patient records confirmed that sleep problems were noted by physicians from various disciplines, but they were not integrated into the clinical assessment with a structured approach, despite providing symptomatic pharmaceutical, behavioural, and occupational treatment for the children's sleep problems [1, 25]. Delays in completing formalized sleep assessments were noted, with delays ranging from less than a year to 8 years in our first study [1], but also up to 18 years in clinical everyday practice and in general patients who had

already been prescribed medications affecting their sleep and wake behaviours. Below are some of these behaviours described by parents and/or caregivers:

Oh he - it's like his brain didn't turn on when you woke him up. It's just like automatically he'll forget when he's in the shower the soap; he won't brush his teeth; he forgets his shoes on his way out the door to school; he forgets his backpack; he forgets his lunch; he forgets… It's just like his brain didn't turn on when he woke up. Just like when you wake up, you think I gotta do this, this and this during the day… (Ipsiroglu et al. [1])

… Because then if he has a good night's sleep, he's cheerful:, he's cooperative:, he's pleasant to be around (.) then ((inaudible)) fun, it's great to be around him when he wakes up. When he's not had enough sleep, he's just the total opposite child, it's just like night and day almost. You know, you get this kid that hasn't had enough sleep and is grumpy, he doesn't listen and then he also has a hard time at school. It's-that's the days that we find that he has had an outburst at school, or hasn't gotten along with the kids at school, hasn't done his work at school … … big temper tantrum!!! (Ipsiroglu et al. [1])

…. and he-his head will be at awkward strange angles to the point where sometimes I will even like, remove a pillow from under his head so that he can-it just looks better for me, ((laughs)) like letting him [sleep]… …Like this. (.) Or like this even. ((chuckles)) Like it's really weird angles, way far back and seem to be draped over things. … ((chuckles)) With his butt in the air (.) is probably the weirdest one and he's fast asleep. Just with his thumbs in the air like he's kneeling. (Ipsiroglu et al. [1])

Implications for Best Practice in the Community: To unravel challenging/disruptive sleep/wake behaviours, use a bidirectional explorative communication strategy. This will help to develop a shared language. To understand clinical presentations from the parents' point of view and to give parents a voice, use the modified semi-structured screening concept of BEARS [34] and implement BEARS at the first interview. Parents can fill out BEARS using their own words [35]. Encourage parents to elaborate about their perceptions of "stressful situations" and "restorative sleep" in short accounts that relate to the well-being of the child (and themselves) before they come to the clinic.

2.5 Structured Observations

2.5.1 Sleep-Disordered Breathing

In our first study, functional sleep/wake behaviours assessments revealed that 30% (8/27) of the children with a prenatal alcohol exposure (Foetal Alcohol Spectrum Disorder, FASD diagnosis) had signs of SDB [1]. In our second FASD study, this figure increased to 95% (38/40) with 68% (27/40) showing signs of upper airway narrowing due to adenoids and/or anatomical facial features [51]. In a third study investigating familial WED/RLS in children with various neurodevelopmental and/or neuropsychiatric conditions and their mothers, 93% (26/28) of children and 54%

(15/28) of mothers displayed symptoms [25]. All these diagnoses caused systematic efforts and specific actions (e.g. prescription of mometasone furoate, referral to ear-nose-throat specialist or to the sleep lab), and they also reveal that the capacity to reduce co-morbidities and optimize individual well-being had been missed or focused upon insufficiently. This situation seems to mirror a systemic neglect of sleep problems in our healthcare system [52].

The difference between categorical and functional diagnosis became evident in our Down Syndrome Needs Study, which was conducted in 2015, in collaboration with the Down Syndrome Research Foundation [53]. Individuals with Down syndrome are considered to be one of the high-risk populations for disturbed sleep; in childhood, prevalence rates of SDB are as high as 50% [54], and these rates increase in adulthood to more than 90% [55]. Interestingly, the Down Syndrome Needs Survey revealed that SDB, as a categorical diagnosis, was given to 19% (59/311) of surveyed individuals; however, 85% ($n = 222/261$) had one or a combination of primary SDB symptoms, mainly mouth breathing (59%), snoring (54%), restless sleep (43%), observed breathing pauses (30%), and gasping during sleep (16%). These symptoms had not been investigated before, and thus opportunities for interventions and treatment of SDB symptoms were missed.

Implications for Best Practice in the Community: The first major achievement was describing and discussing facial features with patients/parents as a high-risk factor for SDB and as a frequent cause of challenging/disruptive sleep and wake behaviours, intractable insomnia, and ADHD-like behaviours, respectively.

2.5.2 WED/RLS

Twenty-eight paediatric patients with early-onset and intractable chronic insomnia and neurodevelopmental and/or neuropsychiatric conditions, as well as their mothers, were assessed at a sleep/wake behaviours clinic. In addition to clinical assessments, structured behavioural observations were obtained during a SCIT [25]. All patients fulfilled the criteria for circadian sleep/wake rhythm disorders, 50% had reported parasomnias, and 20/28 presented with signs of sleep-disordered breathing. In order to examine a patient population with familial WED/RLS, we focused only on patients whose mothers had been previously diagnosed with WED/RLS ($n = 28/31$). Quotations from parents illustrated the experienced clinical symptoms from a narrative-based perspective. The formal and informal SCIT-related information was positive in all cases. Formal test: 17 (61%) participated actively in the formal test; 16/17 (94%) patients reported various descriptions of their urge to move and showed signs of involuntary movements of legs/feet/toes. Only one patient (treated with clonidine 0.1 mg/daily at night-time) who was previously diagnosed with parasomnia and an anxiety disorder (treated with fluoxetine mgs/daily) in our cohort did not show/report motor signs and sensory discomfort during the formal test. In the remaining 11 (39%) cases, patients could not participate actively in the test; therefore, the observation-based involuntary motor movements at random rest situations were utilized as an informal test from the reports. Sensory processing abnormalities were stratified based on the types of parental reports and observations, all patients presented with various sensory processing abnormalities: 96% ($n = 27$) had a tactile sensitivity, 69% ($n = 20$) presented with a shifted pain threshold, and auditory, visual, and/or oral sensitivities were reported in 21% ($n = 6$) of the patients.

Implications for Best Practice in the Community: The SCIT, as applied in functional sleep/wake behaviours assessments, enabled the structured, observational assessment of the first three self-reported criteria that are essential for diagnosis: (1) an urge to move the legs, usually accompanied by uncomfortable or unpleasant sensations in the legs; (2) symptoms begin or worsen during periods of rest; and (3) symptoms are partially or totally relieved by movement. This way the discussion of the 4th essential WED/RLS criteria (i.e. symptoms occur mainly in the evening/night) and 5th criteria (i.e. differential diagnoses: symptoms cannot be solely accounted by another medical condition) was also cued in a structured way. In addition, the SCIT lays a foundation of shared understanding between patients/families/caregivers and professionals.

2.6 Conclusion and Solutions

Analysis of professionals' systematic inattention to the sequelae of sleep problems revealed that this practice was due to an insufficient understanding of the interconnections between night-time problems and daytime behaviours. The awareness is present but training is missing (i.e. the interviewed physician shared the statement: *I was not formally trained to address sleep problems* [1]). This testimonial reveals a culture of separation between *practically experienced* and *academically learned knowledge* when it comes to making clinical decisions. Interpretations of sleep-related symptoms and decision-making in clinical practice are negatively impacted by *categorical diagnoses* and the complexity of situations in which these diagnoses present; therefore, symptoms are not well-understood, and the expectations from involved parties (e.g. parents) might bias further understanding. From a public health perspective, appropriate diagnosis and treatment of sleep problems might prevent medication prescription cascades that children and youth with neurodevelopmental and/or neuropsychiatric conditions often experience, causing iatrogenic harm in children with complex neurobehavioural symptomatology, as we have previously observed and reported. Many children referred to our clinic had previously received child psychiatry/mental health diagnoses, which were partly or completely resolved after treatment of the underlying cause of their sleep problems [43, 44].

2.6.1   Solution I: *Parents as Partners*

Implications for Best Practice in the Community: Upon analysing the communication deficits and optimizing our understanding about various perceptions and knowledge in regard to challenging/disruptive sleep/wake behaviours, we adapted the concept of explorational history taking and developed together a plot (therapeutic emplotment) as a shared language strategy in our clinical setting.

Feedback from a non-governmental organization advocating for patient rights highlighted that the conventional reporting method was perceived as unidirectional and thus inefficient. In response to this feedback, we started to address parents directly in all reports. This change reflects that parents are acknowledged in the reports as *first-line treatment providers and partners*. Furthermore, the commitment to present the symptoms that parents had reported in their own words was fulfilled by incorporating direct quotations into the reports and implementing *a patient-based quality assurance strategy*. After a very short period of time, it became clear that parents and assessing professionals were describing (for the first time in many cases) the same phenomena (many of which were not well-recognized by the assessing physician) using a shared language. In this manner, assessing physicians and parents collaboratively explored presentations and dimensions of the intractable sleep problem of their child. In consequence, we developed assessment forms, which capture parents' descriptions of behaviours and activities, as well as quotations of clinically relevant descriptive features of sleep and wake behaviours [56, 57].

The use of plain and transparent language to describe patients' behaviours and patient/family interactions avoids inaccessible medical terminology, is perceived by parents as *respectful*, and increased adherence. Sentences about parents are started by using their names (never refer to them in third person, as *he* or *she*, and always address parents/caregivers by their last names) and avoided language that has negative implications or is disrespectful (e.g. *he denies that his daughter snores*) toward parents/caregivers. Hence, the reports became a document of shared understanding adding the concept of plot development to the foundational framework of our clinic.

2.6.2   Solution II: *Structuring Assessments in the Community*

In an atmosphere of economic constraints, protected space for discussions between physicians and other healthcare professionals is scarce. When educating physicians, we often refer to paediatric sleep research and must convince the referring physician that considering the underlying cause of the sleep problem as a primary cause of disease might reverse mental health diagnoses such as ADHD [43] and/or as autism

[44]. Autism *alone* might not explain the challenging and disruptive behaviours, and in fact, an underlying sleep problem, such as WED/RLS, might cause stereotypical repetitive discomfort or pain-associated behaviours (e.g. stomping with the feet or kicking walls). In other words, in patients with ASD and intractable insomnia, WED/RLS can cause discomfort and/or pain, and the effects of sleep deprivation contribute to the challenging and disruptive daytime behaviours and are treatable.

Implications for Best Practice in the Community: The second stage of our clinical research aimed to find ways to expand the clinical understanding of sleep problems in children with neurodevelopmental and neuropsychiatric conditions, in collaboration with their parents/caregivers. With increasing understanding, parents/caregivers and physicians started to challenge categorical daytime-based diagnoses, which had been given without assessing possible underlying sleep problems.

References

1. Ipsiroglu OS, McKellin WH, Carey N, Loock C. "They silently live in terror …" Why sleep problems and night-time related quality-of-life are missed in children with a fetal alcohol spectrum disorder. Soc Sci Med. 2013;79:76–83. https://doi.org/10.1016/j.socscimed.2012.10.027.
2. Ethnography [Def. 1]. (n.d.). In Oxford Dictionaries. Accessed on July 4, 2015, from http://www.oxforddictionaries.com/definition/english/ethnography.
3. Kleinman A. The illness narratives: suffering, healing, and the human condition. New York, NY: Basic Books; 1988.
4. Kleinman A. Catastrophe and caregiving: the failure of medicine as an art. Lancet. 2008;371(9606):22–3.
5. Ecology [Def. 1]. (n.d.). In Oxford Dictionaries. Accessed on July 14, 2015, from http://www.oxforddictionaries.com/definition/english/ecology.
6. Lucyshyn J, Albin R. Comprehensive support to families of children with disabilities and problem behaviors: keeping it "friendly". In: Singer G, Powers L, editors. Families, disabilities, and empowerment: active coping skills and strategies for family interventions. Baltimore, MD: Paul H Brookes; 1993. p. 365–407.
7. Lucyshyn J, Albin R, Nixon C. Embedding comprehensive behavioural support in family ecology: an experimental single-case analysis. J Consult Clin Pyschol. 1997;65:241–51.
8. McKellin W. Hearing impaired families: the social ecology of hearing loss. Soc Sci Med. 1995;40(11):1469–80.
9. Dickens C. The pickwick papers. London: Chapman & Hall; 1837.
10. American Academy of Sleep Medicine Task Force. Sleep-related breathing disorders in adults: recommendations for syndrome definition and measurement techniques in clinical research. The Report of an American Academy of Sleep Medicine Task Force. Sleep. 1999;1(22):667–89.
11. Epstein L, Kristo D, Strollo P, Friedman N, Malhotra A, Patil S, et al. Clinical guideline for the evaluation, management and long-term care of obstructive sleep apnea in adults. J Clin Sleep Med. 2009;5(3):263–76.
12. Mindell JA, Owens JA. A clinical guide to pediatric sleep: diagnosis and management of sleep problems. 2nd ed. Philadelphia, PA: Lippincott Williams & Wilkins; 2009.

13. Jan JE, Owens JA, Weiss M, Johnson K, Wasdell M, Freeman R, Ipsiroglu OS. Sleep hygiene for children with neurodevelopmental disabilities. Paediatrics. 2008;122(6):1343–50. https://doi.org/10.1542/peds.2007-3308.
14. Jan JE, Asante KO, Conry JL, Fast DK, Bax MC, Ipsiroglu OS, et al. Sleep health issues for children with FASD: Clinical considerations. Int J Pediatr. 2010;2010:639048. https://doi.org/10.1155/2010/639048.
15. Malow BA, Byars K, Johnson K, Weiss S, Bernal P, Goldman S, et al. A practice pathway for the identification, evaluation, and management of insomnia in children and adolescents with autism spectrum disorders. Pediatrics. 2012;130(Suppl. 2):S106–24. https://doi.org/10.1542/peds.2012-0900I.
16. Wiggs L, Stores G. Severe sleep disturbance and daytime challenging behaviour in children with severe learning disabilities. J Intellect Disabil Res. 1996;40(6):518–28.
17. Zucconi M, Bruni O. Sleep disorders in children with neurologic diseases. Semin Pediatr Neurol. 2001;8(4):258–75.
18. Chervin RD. Sleepiness, fatigue, tiredness, and lack of energy in obstructive sleep apnea. Chest. 2000;118(2):372–9. https://doi.org/10.1378/chest.118.2.372.
19. Gottlieb DJ, Vezina RM, Chase C, Lesko SM, Heeren TC, Weese-Mayer DE, et al. Symptoms of sleep-disordered breathing in 5-year-old children are associated with sleepiness and problem behaviors. Pediatrics. 2003;112(4):870–7.
20. Johnson K, Malow BA. Sleep in children with autism spectrum disorders. Curr Treat Options Neurol. 2008;10(5):350–9. https://doi.org/10.1007/s11940-008-0038-5.
21. Ferber R. Solve your child's sleep problems: new, revised, and expanded edition. New York, NY: Touchstone; 2006.
22. Jan JE, Bax M, Owens JA, Ipsiroglu OS, Wasdell M. Neurophysiology of circadian rhythm sleep disorders of children with neurodevelopmental disabilities. Eur J Pediatr Neurol. 2012;16(5):403–12. https://doi.org/10.1016/j.ejpn.2012.01.002.
23. Picchietti DL, Bruni O, de Weerd A, Durmer JS, Kotagal S, Owens JA, et al. Pediatric restless legs syndrome diagnostic criteria: an update by the International Restless Legs Syndrome Study Group. Sleep Med. 2013;14(12):1253–9. https://doi.org/10.1016/j.sleep.2013.08.778.
24. Coccagna G, Vetrugno R, Lombardi C, Provini F. Restless legs syndrome: an historical note. Sleep Med. 2004;5(3):27–283. https://doi.org/10.1016/j.sleep.2004.01.002.
25. Ipsiroglu OS, Beyzaei N, Berger M, Wagner A, Dhalla S, Garden J, Stockler S. "Emplotted narratives" and structured "behavioral observations" supporting the diagnosis of Willis-Ekbom disease/restless legs syndrome in children with neurodevelopmental conditions. CNS Neurosci Ther. 2016;22(11):894–905. https://doi.org/10.1111/cns.12564.
26. Wiggs L, Stores G. Sleep disturbance in children and adolescents with disorders of development: its significance and management. Oxford: Cambridge University Press; 2001.
27. Wiggs L, Stores G. Sleep patterns and sleep disorders in children with autistic spectrum disorders: insights using parent report and actigraphy. Dev Med Child Neurol. 2004;46(6):372–80. https://doi.org/10.1017/S0012162204000611.
28. Gruber R, Wise MS, Frenette S, Knäauper B, Boom A, Fontil L, Carrier J. The association between sleep spindles and IQ in healthy school-age children. Int J Psychophysiol. 2013;89(2):229–40. https://doi.org/10.1016/j.ijpsycho.2013.03.018.
29. Sivertsen B, Posserud M, Gillberg C, Lundervold A, Hysing M. Sleep problems in children with autism spectrum problems: a longitudinal population-based study. Autism. 2012;16(2):139–50. https://doi.org/10.1177/1362361311404255.
30. Wolfson AR, Montgomery-Downs H, editors. The Oxford handbook of infant, child, and adolescent sleep and behaviour. New York, NY: Oxford University Press; 2013.
31. Sloper T, Beresford B. Families with disabled children - social and economic needs are high but remain largely unmet. BMJ. 2006;333(7575):928–9. https://doi.org/10.1136/bmj.39017.633310.BE.

32. Krakowiak P, Goodlin-Jones B, Hertz-Picciotto I, Croen L, Hansen R. Sleep problems in children with autism spectrum disorders, developmental delays, and typical development: A population-based study. J Sleep Res. 2008;17:197–206. https://doi.org/10.1111/j.1365-2869.2008.00650.x.
33. Ipsiroglu OS. Applying ethnographic methodologies & ecology to unveil dimensions of sleep problems in children & youth with neurodevelopmental conditions (Doctoral dissertation). Vancouver, BC: University of British Columbia; 2016.
34. Owens JA, Dalzell V. Use of the BEARS sleep screening tool in a pediatric residents continuity clinic: a pilot study. Sleep Med. 2005;6:63–9. https://doi.org/10.1016/j.sleep.2004.07.015.
35. Ipsiroglu OS, Carey N, Collet J, Fast D, Garden J, Jan JE, et al. De- medicalizing sleep: sleep assessment tools in the community setting for clients (patients) with FASD & prenatal substance exposure. National Organisation for Fetal Alcohol Syndrome – UK (NOFAS-UK): Fetal Alcohol Forum. 2012. Accessed on May 1, 2015, from http://www.nofas-uk.org/PDF/FETAL%20ALCOHOL%20FORUM%20Issue%207%20June%202012.pdf.
36. Stockler S, Moeslinger D, Herle M, Wimmer B, Ipsiroglu OS. Cultural aspects in the management of inborn errors of metabolism. J Inherit Metab Dis. 2012;35(6):1147–53. https://doi.org/10.1007/s10545-012-9455-4.
37. Bruni O, Fabrizi P, Ottaviano S, Cortesi F, Giannotti F, Guidetti V. Prevalence of sleep disorders in childhood and adolescence with headache: a case-control study. Cephalalgia. 1997;17(4):492–8.
38. Chervin RD, Hedger K, Dillon JE, Pituch KJ. Pediatric sleep questionnaire (PSQ): Validity and reliability of scales for sleep-disordered breathing, snoring, sleepiness, and behavioral problems. Sleep Med. 2000;1(1):21–32.
39. Cicourel A. Hearing is not believing: language and the structure of belief in medical communication. In: Fisher S, Todd AD, editors. The social organization of doctor-patient communication. Washington, DC: Center for Applied Linguistics; 1983. p. 221–39.
40. Fontana A, Frey J. The interview. From structured questions to negotiated text. In: Denzin NK, Lincoln YS, editors. Handbook of qualitative research. 2nd ed. Thousand Oaks, CA: Sage Publications; 2000. p. 645–72.
41. Bruni O, Ottaviano S, Guidetti V, Romoli M, Innocenzi M, Cortesi F, Giannotti F. The Sleep Disturbance Scale for Children (SDSC) - construction and validation of an instrument to evaluate sleep disturbances in childhood and adolescence. J Sleep Res. 1996;5(4):251–61.
42. Owens JA, Spirito A, McGuinn M. The Children's Sleep Habits Questionnaire (CSHQ): psychometric properties of a survey instrument for school aged children. Sleep. 2000;23(8):1043–51.
43. Ipsiroglu OS, Berger M, Lin T, Elbe D, Stockler S, Carleton B. Pathways to overmedication and polypharmacy: case examples from adolescents with fetal alcohol spectrum disorders. In: Di Pietro N, Illes J, editors. The science and ethics of antipsychotic use in children. Waltham, MA: Elsevier; 2015a. p. 125–48.
44. Ipsiroglu OS. Autismus-Spektrum-Störungen und Willis-Ekbom-Erkrankung. Ein Plädoyer für explorative Anamnesen [Autism spectrum disorders and Willis Ekbom disease. A plea for explorative histories]. In: Paditz E, Sauseng W, editors. Schlafmedizin Kompendium [Sleep Medicine Compendium]. Dresden: Kleanthes; 2015.
45. Malow BA, Connolly HV, Weiss SK, Halbower A, Goldman S, Hyman SL, et al. The pediatric sleep clinical global impressions scale-a new tool to measure pediatric insomnia in autism spectrum disorders. J Dev Behav Pediatr. 2016;37(5):370–6. https://doi.org/10.1097/DBP.0000000000000307.
46. Robinson A, Malow B. Gabapentin shows promise in treating pediatric insomnia. Sleep. 2012;35:A394. https://doi.org/10.1177/0883073812463069.
47. American Academy of Sleep Medicine. International classification of sleep disorders, revised: Diagnostic and coding manual. Chicago, IL: American Academy of Sleep Medicine; 2001.
48. Picchietti M, Picchietti D. Advances in pediatric restless legs syndrome: iron, genetics, diagnosis and treatment. Sleep Med. 2010;11:643–51. https://doi.org/10.1016/j.sleep.2009.11.014.
49. Todd A, Fisher S. The social organization of doctor-patient communication. Norwood, NJ: Ablex Publishing; 1993.

50. Ipsiroglu OS, Andrew G, Carmichael-Olson H, Chen M, Collet J, Pei J, et al. How to approach sleep problems in children with FASD: the 1st Canadian FASD & SLEEP consensus paper. J Populat Ther Clin Pharmacol. 2011;18(3):422–3.
51. Ipsiroglu OS, Wind K, Hung Y-H, Berger M, Chan F, Yu W, et al. Prenatal alcohol exposure and sleep-wake behaviors: exploratory and naturalistic observations in the clinical setting and in an animal model. Sleep Med. 2019;54:101–12. https://doi.org/10.1016/j.sleep.2018.10.006. Epub 2018 Oct 25. PMID: 30530254.
52. Ipsiroglu OS, Jan JE, Freeman RD, Laswick A, Milner R, Mitton C, et al. How to approach pediatric sleep in British Columbia: a consensus paper. B C Med J. 2009;50(9):512–6.
53. Ipsiroglu OS, Beyzaei N, Tse E, Marwaha A. [BC Down syndrome survey results – sleep/wake behaviours: sleep diagnoses]. Unpublished raw data presented at the Sleep Summit Meeting at the Down Syndrome Research Foundation, Vancouver, BC. 2015b, June. Accessed on August 17, 2015, from http://www.dsrf.org/media/BCDSS%20%20Focus%20Group%20Discussion%20(Final)%20-%20June%205,%202015.pdf.
54. Stores G, Stores R. Sleep disorders and their clinical significance in children with Down syndrome. Dev Med Child Neurol. 2013;55(2):126–30. https://doi.org/10.1111/j.1469-8749.2012.04422.x.
55. Lal C, White DR, Joseph JE, van Bakergem K, LaRose A. Sleep-disordered breathing in Down syndrome. Chest. 2015;147(2):570–9. https://doi.org/10.1378/chest.14-0266.
56. Mattingly C. The concept of therapeutic 'emplotment'. Soc Sci Med. 1994;38(6):811–22.
57. Mattingly C. Healing dramas and clinical plots: the narrative structure of experience. Cambridge: Cambridge University Press; 1998.

Craniofacial Growth and Development

3

German O. Ramirez-Yañez

3.1 Introduction

All human beings are born with the potential of growing and developing between normal patterns, with the exception of those born with a congenital syndrome or a genetic disorder. The pioneers in orthodontics described normal growth as achieving the best proportions of the mouth in a good relation with the other structures of the craniofacial system, maintaining a balance between them, and permitting each tooth to occupy its normal position [1, 2]. Such a statement is currently supported by insights on neurobiology and epigenetics [3–5]. So, the first question regarding the etiology of malocclusions is: are they genetically or environmentally induced?

A strong controversy still is on the table on that matter. At the beginning of last century, some authors defended that craniofacial growth and development was genetically driven and, the only possibility of variation in the mouth was changing the position of the teeth [6]. Such theory postulated that craniofacial growth occurs exclusively by bone remodeling. It did not consider any role for other structures, such as sutures, cranial base synchondrosis, the mandibular condylar cartilage, or muscular loading on the craniofacial bones [7]. Later, Moss proposed the functional matrix theory [8]. He theorized the size and shape of the maxillaries are determined by the functional matrices [8–12]. That plus the advent of new theories, including the cybernetic theory [13, 14], which causes a division where some authors dispute craniofacial growth is driven by genetics, while others argue it is led by function. The most recent developments in that field are showing that both sides may be in some way correct. Neither genetics alone nor function per se has the steering control. It appears to be genetics guided by function/environment which leads craniofacial growth and development. In other words, genetics is expressed accordingly to the functional demands.

G. O. Ramirez-Yañez (✉)
Private Practice, Aurora Kids Dentistry, Aurora, ON, Canada

© Springer Nature Switzerland AG 2019
E. Liem (ed.), *Sleep Disorders in Pediatric Dentistry*,
https://doi.org/10.1007/978-3-030-13269-9_3

To understand that, it is important to remember that the craniofacial complex is composed by various tissues, which contain a matrix and cells. Currently, there is enough knowledge to understand that cell's biology is controlled by the constantly changing environment and not by its genes [15]. An environmental stimulus on the cells modifies cytoplasmic processes altering gene expression. In that context, such stimulus influences cell movement, control cell survival, or even determine when a cell should die [16, 17]. All those phenomena are explained by epigenetics, which has helped the scientific community to understand the critical control of cell and tissue differentiation. It has also provided a better understanding of the complexities of craniofacial growth and development [3, 4, 18].

3.2   Craniofacial Growth and Development Driven by Epigenetics: A New Theory

A theory in modern science refers to a well-confirmed type of explanation of phenomenon. Several theories of craniofacial growth and development have been postulated in the past, but none of them have fully explained that phenomenon, as they have based their arguments on either genetics or function. Today, it needs to be revised under the current knowledge of epigenetics.

Epigenetics is the science of how environmental signals select, modify, and regulate gene activity. It studies the molecular mechanisms by which environment controls gene activity [15, 19, 20]. Cells process thousands of signals from the surrounding environment. In that way, cells determine the appropriate biological responses to ensure their survival [21, 22]. Genes contained in any cell in the body are not able to self-regulate their expression. When a gene product is needed, a signal from the environment activates the expression of that gene [23].

Today the scientific community has revealed the human genome, while the human epigenome is still under study. It is known that every gene, which is a DNA chain, is wrapped by a structure named the histone. Besides the histone, there are some small structures which are the epigenomes. They activate the histone, and so, the gene can be wrapped or unwrapped. In other words, the gene can be activated or deactivated [24]. That interaction can analogically be explained as the epigenome being the switch which may turn a light bulb on or off.

Thus, the next question is: who provide the information to the epigenomes to switch on or off a gene? The answer is: the environment. The epigenome acts as a link between the environment and the genes. It determines when a gene should produce or stop producing certain substance by the cells. In that way, the system is modified and adapts to environmental changes. So, the epigenome is sensing what is happening in the environment to modify the genetic expression [15].

For example, it has been demonstrated that only 5% of cancer and cardiovascular diseases are inherited [25] and a significant cases of cancer in humans are induced by environmental alterations and not by defective genes [26–28]. Is the current knowledge in epigenetics showing orthodontics that something similar may occur with malocclusions?

It is generally accepted that malocclusions are a developmental problem highly influenced by genes' expression. Most biological dysfunctions start at the level of cell's molecules and ions. Knowing that cell biology can be modified by the environment, it can be argued that it is possible to modify the cell biology in the craniofacial complex to improve or disrupt the cells' function. It is also valid to argue that at birth the environment start playing a critical role in determining genes' expression in the cells found in the craniofacial tissues. Thus, every human being has the potential to grow and develop within normal or abnormal patterns. The environment to which a newborn is exposed (e.g., habits, correct or incorrect oral functions, correct or incorrect breathing pathway, diet, etc.) is going to determine the expression of the cells and so, how tissues develop and mature.

When a baby is born the genome is waiting for the epigenome to sense the environment and determine how the genes should express. Regarding to craniofacial growth and development, if the baby's mouth is exposed to an ideal environment, the epigenome will switch "on" certain genes and keep "off" others to produce a normal growth and development of the maxillaries [5]. Conversely, when baby's mouth is exposed to an unnatural environment (e.g., bottle-feeding instead of breastfeeding), the epigenome switches on or off the required genes adapting the system to that unnatural situation [29, 30]. Thus, at crucial moments of facial development, very small fluctuations can result in either of two very different types of occlusal relationship [31].

The genetic influence on malocclusion's development has been supported by arguing children exhibit the same type of malocclusion to that one or both parents may have. Under the umbrella of epigenetics, it can be argued back that the parents replicated a similar environment for the child to that they had when they grew up. That environment (e.g., similar diet, habits and posture mimicking, etc.) produces an effect in the cells' biology of the child, who will resemble the facial appearance of the parents [32]. Another argument against is the evidence demonstrating that rural populations significantly increase the incidence of malocclusions within one generation after moving to urban areas [33–35]. Figure 3.1 shows how environmental changes may be associated with deviation of the normal pathway and how correcting the oral functions may bring craniofacial growth and development into a more physiological pathway.

On the other hand, when a malocclusion has already established, it is valid to argue that such a change in the environmental conditions would continue modifying the cells' biology in the craniofacial complex (e.g., lack of growth and development of the jaws). By directly treating the cause of the malocclusion, the dysfunctions, better results could be achieved. Up today, science has not elucidated how to do that directly by targeting the cells with a particular substance. However, there is scientific evidence demonstrating that by modifying wrong patterns in the environment (e.g., oral dysfunctions, tongue posture, mode of breathing, etc.), it is possible to improve the biological response at the craniofacial complex [36–38].

Therefore, craniofacial growth and development must be considered driven neither by genetics nor by function but by the epigenome. It interprets the environmental

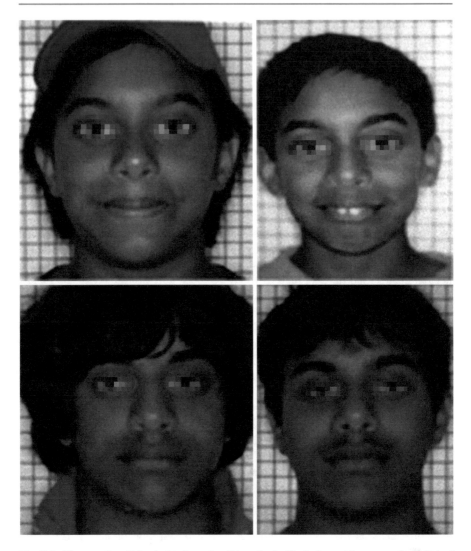

Fig. 3.1 Photographs of identical twins, who did not look alike before as the one on the right had altered oral functions and his craniofacial growth and development proceeded in a different pathway compared to his twin brother. After correcting the oral functions, they look more alike. Photographs presented with permission from the patients and Dr. Chris Farrell

conditions and switches "on/off" the genetic expression accordingly [5, 15, 19, 20, 24, 36, 37]. Today's scientific knowledge permits to say craniofacial growth and development is determined by both genetics and environment, with epigenetics acting as a modulator. That phenomenon occurs during the human life spam. Based on that knowledge, it can be postulated that when a deviation from the normal developmental pattern is observed or diagnosed, it can be reversed to normality by changing the environment, unless a congenital/genetic defect is involved.

As the environment changes in the craniofacial system, the epigenomes sense those changes and modulate genes' expression. At an early developmental stage, when the cells are less differentiated and growth potential is still optimal, it would be easier to bring the system into a normal pattern of growth and development. At that moment, the environmental influences may produce better effects in genes' expression, modifying tissue development and maturation. Thus, the best time for the environment to exert the most positive effect on craniofacial growth and development would be at the first years of life, when all oral functions and the breathing pattern are imprinted in the brain, as well as when the highest growth potential is at the jaws [39–41].

Epigenetics also explain what is generally accepted today: bone growth is stimulated by the activity of the muscles [42, 43]. In a newborn, the muscular system in the head and neck needs to further develop in order to produce the correct loading on the craniofacial bones [44]. That stimulates both, endochondral and intramembranous ossifications in the mandible and the maxilla [43]. Then, both of them can reach an ideal size and shape for the teeth accommodating later. So, guiding craniofacial growth and development through stimulating correct muscular activity since the first day of life is critical. To achieve that, correct breastfeeding is an asset to stimulate muscular growth of the masticatory and facial muscles, that initiate a cascade of events, such as: (1) both, the maxilla and the mandible are properly loaded by the muscles (environment), (2) epigenomes in the oral system recognize that load (epigenetics), (3) the required genes for tissue growth and development are activated (genetics), and (4) all that lead to an ideal size and shape of the maxilla and the mandible, which in turn produces enough space for the erupting teeth (outcome). In that context, breastfeeding becomes one of the milestones when considering the causes of malocclusion. However, it is not only encouraging breastfeeding. It has to be performed under certain considerations as explained later on this chapter to produce the best outcome.

3.3 The Importance of Breastfeeding on Craniofacial Growth and Development

Several human functions are developed during the first years of life, with three of them being critical for craniofacial growth and development: breathing, swallowing, and mastication. This section approaches craniofacial growth and development since birth from a different point of view to that considered in the traditional books, where growth and development of the mineralized tissues is the major focus.

The first premise proposed is that all human beings are born to have an ideal size of the dental arches, which permits a correct position of the teeth. Therefore, any unnatural behavior occurring during the first days of life starts a deviation in the breathing pattern and/or oral functions. That then initiates a cascade of events ending in a malocclusion. In that context, breastfeeding, the first function performed in all mammals, has to be in a correct and natural way [45], as it is the base for the development of a correct breathing, swallowing, and masticatory pattern, and so, producing an appropriate stimulus on the craniofacial complex [46, 47].

3.3.1   Breastfeeding and Breathing

At birth, all human beings are premeditated to be nasal breathers [48]. The posterior part of the mouth is the entrance of the oropharynx, which is the conduit for two separated functions, swallowing and respiration. Over the first months of life, the entrance of the oropharynx, at the back of the mouth, is partially closed at the midline by the uvula and the epiglottis which are in a close proximity [48]. The sides of that entrance to the oropharynx remain open permitting the passage of the breast milk. In human infants, as in other mammals, swallowing and respiration should occur simultaneously [49–51]. In that context, the newborn can attach to the breast, maintain suction, and nibble mom's breast to get the milk and swallow it while breathing through the nose. The breast's nipple is hold between the palate and tongue, while the milk is extracted from the breast by sagittal movements of the mandible, with the lips sealing the mouth around the mom's breast. In that way, the newborn learns how to breathe through the nose while milk passes through the mouth and reaches the lateral openings at the back of the mouth. In other words, nasal breathing is performed together with swallowing [40].

To perform the three functions (suction, swallowing, and breathing) without either one affecting the others, the baby has to be in a correct position. That permits the passage of air through the nose while the milk passes through the mouth. To achieve that, the newborn has to be fed in a semi-seated position and not lying down [45]. A wrong position can deviate the oral functions from a normal pattern and inappropriately stimulate growth in the various components of the oral system. Furthermore, it increases the risk of habits [46, 47].

Breathing is a primal function necessary for survival. Human beings are obligate nasal breathers, and the mouth is a backup organ for this function. The passage of air through the nose will create an airflow into the nose and the nasopharynx, which stimulates development of the nasal cavity [52–55]. The palate is at the same time the floor of the nose and the roof of the mouth. Airflow pushes down the floor of the nose, modeling and remodeling the maxilla and palatal bones [52, 53]. That force pushing downward is counteracted by the force delivered by the tongue on the palate holding the nipple. In such a situation, there are two counter-directional forces: one on the nasal aspect of the palate pushing downward and another on the oral aspect of the palate pushing upward. When two forces are delivered in an opposite vertical direction, the resultant force expresses toward the sides (Fig. 3.2).

Thus, a newborn breathing through the nose, properly breastfeeding, and swallowing with no obstruction stimulates transverse development of the maxilla [56]. A natural palatal expansion occurs with breastfeeding, and the newborn learns to breathe through the nose [40, 56, 57]. That makes more room for the tongue and facilitates the development of a healthy nasal airway [57]. In this way, the maxilla reaches its maximum transverse development, which is expected to be about 90% of its total size at the end of infancy [58, 59].

An improper position of the newborn during breastfeeding (e.g., lying down or bottle-feeding) does not produce the same stimuli on transverse maxillary development. A newborn lying down at breastfeeding, a common position for

Fig. 3.2 Airflow pushes the palate down, whereas tongue pressures upward. The resultant force toward the sides stimulating transverse development of the maxilla

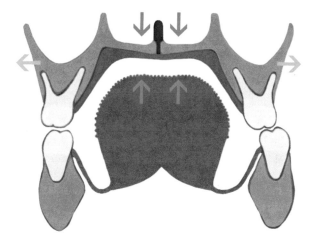

bottle-feeding, has to descend the tongue as it moves backward by gravity. That reduces the space in the oropharynx [60]. In such a position, the mom's breast may cover the nostrils and block the entrance of air through the nose. Still the newborn can extract the milk from the breast in a similar way as described above, holding the breast's nipple with the tongue against the palate. However, the passage of air through the nose is significantly reduced, and the baby has to release mom's breast and open the mouth to catch air. The air comes through the mouth instead of coming through the nose. That pushes the uvula upward and the epiglottis downward opening the entrance of the oropharynx. Breathing through the mouth causes opening that passage before time, as the oropharynx has not developed yet in the new born and, it makes the tissues in the uvula and epiglottis slender. By repetition, the newborn learns to breathe through the mouth instead of the nose, and the tissues at the entrance of the oropharynx become laxer. Even worst, the baby learns how to get air through an unnatural way, the mouth [61, 62].

A newborn fed with a bottle goes through a similar pathway. Besides the effect on the tongue position mentioned above, the bottle's nipple is made of rubber or silicon and does not have the same resistance to deformation as the breast's nipple [63]. In that context, the newborn does not necessarily need to create a great pressure against the palate with the tongue to hold the nipple and extract the milk from the bottle. It means less pressure on the maxilla, which stimulates less development [64, 65]. Even more, the position of the newborn lying down permits the mandible to drop down plus the mouth is not totally sealed by the lips around the bottle's nipple, and so, air can come through the mouth stimulating mouth breathing. Those are key factors in stimulating mouth breathing in a newborn [66, 67].

Therefore, nasal obstruction caused either by mom's breast blocks the nose when the baby is lying down or the lips stay apart because the position of the baby at feeding, causes a cascade of events, such as: air passing through the mouth; the tongue displaces downward permitting the passage of air to the pharynx; tongue descend reduces the upward loading on the palate. It is also followed by a descends of the hyoid bone, which increases the activity of the muscles depressing the mandible, and finally, all of them together increase the risk of developing a malocclusion, such as open bite or crossbite [30, 65, 68].

3.3.2   Breastfeeding and Swallowing

During the first months of life, the baby's diet is liquid. That permits an easy passage of the breast milk through the openings between the pillars at the entrance of the oropharynx [48, 61]. Besides that, the movements of the anterior portion of the tongue holding the nipple against the palate plus the peristaltic movements moving the milk to the back prepare the tongue muscles to perform the right movements during swallowing [69].

At approximately 4–6 months of age, the uvula begins to ascend and the epiglottis descends. As the child grows, the posterior portion of the tongue, throat, and soft palate become the compliant parts of the adult pharynx. Thus, the posterior third of the tongue lies vertically becoming the anterior wall of the pharynx [61].

As discussed above, when a baby is fed with a bottle or wrongly positioned when breastfeeding, generally the baby is lying down. That brings the tongue backward, and it is displaced downward by the bottle nipple. That positions the tongue backward, so pushing the uvula and epiglottis into the oropharynx opening that close contact between them characteristic at the first months of life. Such a situation occurring before the physiological descend of the epiglottis reduces the tonus of the tissues in both the soft palate and epiglottis. Also, the tip of the tongue is not reaching the position at the incisive papilla, an area now being occupied by the bottle's nipple. Then, the tip of the tongue learns to posture close to the lower incisors [66, 70]. In that flatten position, the tongue performs incorrectly when transporting the milk backward, and so, an incorrect swallowing pattern is imprinted in the brain [40].

3.3.3   Breastfeeding and Mastication

During the first years of life, the masticatory muscles grow and develop to reach the right tonus. That allows the mandible to properly perform when harder food becomes part of the diet [69, 71]. The diet during the first year of life is liquid, and at the end of the first year, soft food is introduced to the baby's diet. Finally, semifibrous and fibrous food is added to the infant's diet between the second and third year of life [72].

That transition from liquid to semi-fibrous (hard) diet has an effect on the masticatory, facial, and neck muscles. It stimulates an increase in the number of fibers and the muscular mass [73]. A natural transition in the diet increases the masticatory muscles' strength, which able those muscles to destroy a harder diet when all the primary teeth are erupted [74]. Such an increase in muscular strength means an increase in bone loading, particularly on the maxilla and mandible. A higher loading on the bones produces bone apposition, which leads to maxillary and mandibular growth and development in the five-spatial dimensions [75, 76]. Maxillary growth and development stimulates growth of the bones joining with the maxilla at the facial sutures, leading ultimately to a higher stimulus on craniofacial growth and development [75, 77, 78].

Breastfeeding is also critical for sagittal mandibular growth. It has been reported that the mandible grows approximately 11 mm during the first year of life [39]. That can be associated to the response of the mandible to that forward and backward movements occurring during breastfeeding [14]. An anteroposterior displacement of the mandible creates a pump effect on the retrodiscal pad at the temporomandibular joint, permitting the release of nutrients and substances that stimulate endochondral ossification at the cartilage placed on the mandibular condyle [14, 79, 80].

All newborns have a convex profile due to a small mandible at birth [81]. So far, the author has not seen a newborn with mandibular prognatism or a concave profile. In an ideal situation, the mandible develops during the intrauterine life to a certain size permitting the development of the oral functions. Breastfeeding stimulates mandibular growth in a sagittal direction catching up the mandible with the maxilla so reaching a normal sagittal relationship at an early age [57, 71, 82]. Later, the transition to semi-fibrous diet permits growth and development of both, the maxilla and mandible. That growth is expressed in a sagittal direction maintaining a normal anteroposterior relationship, as well as in a transverse direction creating the space for the primary teeth and establishing a normal dental occlusion at an early age [57, 71, 81].

3.3.4   The Consequences of an Incorrect and/or Absence of Breastfeeding

It definitively calls anybody's attention to learn that among 46 species of mammals, human beings are the only species with significant malocclusions and caries in their teeth (Dr. Peter Emily—Father of Veterinary Medicine). Thus, the obvious questions are: Why those oral problems are a common finding in humans, but not in other mammals? What are we, human beings, doing different to other species to acquire those problems/diseases? Several responses can be brought up: firstly, all mammals breastfeed their inbreeds for a certain period of time [83]; secondly, other mammal species do not have processed food, bottle-feeding, or pacifiers; and, thirdly, other mammal species are fed with food containing the nutritional factors and the physical consistency they require since they are born [84].

Most human newborns have a distal mandibular position [81]. Then, the mandible will grow and catch with maxillary growth through mandibular movements associated with breastfeeding [14, 39]. Simultaneously, a higher muscular activity required to milk the mom's breast invigorates the masticatory muscles and prepares them to destroy harder food in the future when all primary teeth are in the mouth [57, 69]. All of that account to reach a normal anteroposterior relationship between the maxilla and mandible, enough transverse development of the maxillaries, and a correct vertical dimension of the lower third of the face [47].

In that context, it is valid to state that malocclusions start developing at birth. An incorrect breastfeeding or bottle-feeding leads to less increase in the muscular mass of the masticatory muscles [69], which produces less loading of the maxilla and mandible, reducing the amount of growth and development at both, the maxilla and the mandible [29, 69, 82, 85]. Besides that, a reduced volume of air passing through the nose, because part of the air is passing through the mouth, means the pressure delivered to the palate on the nasal side is decreased, and the stimulus on the maxillary transverse development is reduced. The result is a narrow maxilla [57, 86].

On the other hand, bottle-feeding implies a rubber nipple in the mouth. Bottle's nipple is made of rubber or silicone which deforms less than mom's nipple. So, the tongue is displaced downward and does not learn to position in the physiological area at rest, the incisive papillae. A lowered posture of the tongue stimulated by the presence of the bottle's nipple adds to the lack of stimulus for maxillary transverse development. A similar situation occurs when a pacifier is introduced. Although pacifiers have been recommended by pediatricians to prevent sudden infant death, breastfeeding highly reduces its incidence [87–89]. Therefore, a pacifier is not required to prevent that problem when the newborn is being properly breastfed.

Breastfeeding with a correct posture of the baby, resting on mom's lap and holding the breast nipple without blocking the nose, has to be encouraged in all newborns being exclusive during the first 6 months [82, 87–89]. Then, breastfeeding is mixed with a soft diet during the second half of the first year of life. In this way, respiratory problems and malocclusions may be prevented. That proper environment drives the epigenomes to induce a full growing potential in the baby and so, reaching a normal occlusion with a correct craniofacial growth and development.

Thus, about 4 years of age, the child should have a normal anteroposterior relationship between the maxillaries; diastemas between the primary teeth, which infers a good transverse development of the maxilla and mandible; and, an overbite and overjet of approximately 0–1 mm. Such an ideal situation indicates that a good vertical dimension is developing, which increases further with the eruption of the first permanent molars [57, 72, 81]. In that context, the child is able to hold a fibrous/semihard diet maintaining the correct stimulus during the following developmental stages with a correct breathing and swallowing patterns, which accounts for a normal occlusion in the mixed and permanent dentitions [71, 90–92].

3.3.5 The Consequences of an Incorrect Breathing and Swallowing Patterns Established at an Early Age

Mouth breathing is normally associated with dysfunctional/infant swallow [60, 93]. Correct swallowing is characterized by the tongue positioning against the roof of the mouth and propelling the food bolus backward. In the meantime, teeth touch in centric occlusion bracing the head on the spinal column; lips touch and are unstrained; and the head is held in a steady position on the spinal column and does not move. At the same time, the child is breathing through the nose without difficulty [57, 72].

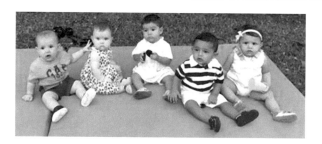

Fig. 3.3 Photographs of infants at their first year of age. The boy at the center of the photograph presents a physiological craniofacial growth and development, whereas the other two boys maintain the mouth open, suggesting mouth breathing. On the other hand, the two girls show lower lip eversion, which may suggest incorrect swallowing

The first signal of mouth breathing is a child with unseal lips at day time or when sleeping, which associates with tongue thrusting (Fig. 3.3). A lower tongue position and mouth breathing become the dominant reflex [40]. The tongue is so displaced backward permitting the passage of air through the mouth; the posterior third of the tongue is displaced backward invading the oropharyngeal area and, therefore, reducing the airway space [60]. The head moves forward, and the hyoid musculature contracts pulling the mandible in a clockwise direction maintaining an open mouth [93]. The muscles of the neck extend and protract the head [94]. All this adaptations occur to maintain an open airway through the mouth in the mouth breather.

Such a change in the muscular activity produces functional changes in the child: the soft palate lies between the tongue and the posterior pharyngeal wall; the tongue is not in contact with the palate on swallowing, so it flattens; scalloped borders appear on the tongue; a greater intermaxillary freeway space is created; swallowing occurs with the teeth in disocclusion [95, 96]; the pressure on the buccal aspects of the posterior teeth delivered by the buccinator muscle increases [97–99]; the palate narrows; and the pharyngeal airway narrows as well, as a result of a lack of transverse development in the maxilla [100]. Furthermore, the posterior teeth tend to extrude, whereas the anterior teeth do not fully erupt producing a different level between the posterior and anterior occlusal planes (Fig. 3.4).

As a mouth-breathing pattern establishes, more functional adaptations occur in the child. A lack of development of the maxilla causes a reduction of the region behind the maxilla (the pterygopalatine and infratemporal fossae), an area occupied by the pterygoid venous plexus. The venous pterygoid plexus receives venous blood from the inferior orbital vein [101]. As the area of the pterygopalatine and infratemporal fossae reduces, the pterygoid venous plexus shrinks, propelling the venous blood back through the inferior orbital vein. It can cause accumulation of venous blood at the inferior region of the eye (purple/dark eye circles) [102, 103].

Another feature of the mouth-breather child is sleep disturbances [104, 105]. A child waking up during the night associates with not reaching the third and/or fourth phase of the sleep [106, 107]. Growth hormone (GH) is released during those sleep phases. So the levels of GH released at night time decreases. That hormonal

Fig. 3.4 Intraoral
photographs of an open bite
patient showing the different
levels between the posterior
and anterior occlusal planes

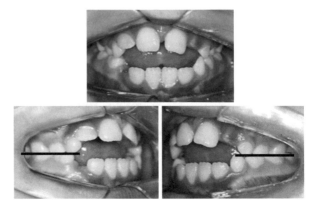

reduction negatively affects craniofacial growth and development, as well as muscular mass development and bone physiology [108–111].

Mouth breathing also stimulates to hold the thumb or any other finger in the mouth to keep it open when the child gets tired [67, 112]. In that situation, the lips are not sealed, and the finger is maintained in the mouth acting as a prop maintaining an oral airway [113]. The presence of the finger in the mouth also increases the inward pressure from the buccinators on swallowing. That pressure can increase up to 10 times at the molar region and up to 40 times at the corner of the mouth [114]. Such a force delivered inwardly with no counteracting force by the tongue, as it is flattened and lowered in mouth breathers, changes the shape of the maxilla making it triangular [115–117].

3.4   Conclusions

Craniofacial growth and development should be comprehended today based on the current scientific evidence. Current knowledge permits to easily understand that the environment plays a definitive role in the expression of the genes contained in the millions of cells composing the various tissues forming the craniofacial complex. In other words, craniofacial growth and development is driven by the interactions between environment and genetics, so epigenetics.

Keeping that in mind, it is important to correct any deviation of the oral functions from birth in order to prevent deviations in craniofacial growth and development. Thus, when a sign (e.g., no spaces in primary dentition, increased overbite and overjet) or symptom (e.g., mouth breathing, incorrect swallowing) is observed in an infant or a child, those should be immediately corrected to re-establish ideal oral functions and bring the craniofacial growth and development into a physiological pathway [30].

Early orthodontics utilizes growth in its favor and early treatment even in primary dentition results in a catch-up of growth [72]. Ideally, maxillary and mandibular growth should be into a normal pattern at 6 years of age when a high percentage of the facial growth has been completed. Delaying treatment up to the pubertal spurt makes treatment more complicated, as the malocclusion does not self-correct with natural growth [118–120]. Therefore, the earlier a deviation from the normal pattern in craniofacial growth and development is detected, the easier to correct and the more stable the results will be [121]. However, the key is focusing in correcting the causes of the problem (e.g., mouth breathing, habits, soft diet, reduced masticatory efforts) and not the consequences (tooth crowding, open bite, deep bite, etc.) [122–124].

The epigenetic theory of craniofacial growth and development presented here calls to establish treatment as early as possible when a sign or symptom of a developing malocclusion is observed in a young child. Today it becomes even more relevant, as it has been established that a deviation in the craniofacial growth and development at an early age can lead to the appearance of temporomandibular dysfunctions later in life [125] or even worse, increasing the risk for pediatric obstructive sleep apnea [126, 127].

References

1. Angle E. The treatment of malocclusion of the teeth, University of California. Philadelphia, PA: White Dental manufacturing Company; 1907.
2. Greene E. The posture of the mandible. Am J Orthod Oral Surg. 1942;28:210–21.
3. Ballestar E. An introduction to epigenetics. Adv Exp Med Biol. 2011;711:1–11.
4. Bayman G, Claes P, Craig J, Goldblatt J, Kung S, Le Souef P, Walters M. Intersections of epigenetics, twinning and developmental asymmetries: insights into monogenic and complex diseases and a role for 3D facial analysis. Twin Res Hum Genet. 2011;14:305–15.
5. Pimenidis M. The neurobiology of orthodontics: treatment of malocclusion through neuroplasticity. Berling: Springer; 2009.
6. Brash J. The aetiology of irregularity and malocclusion of the teeth. London: Dental Board of the United Kingdom; 1929.
7. Carlson D. Theories of craniofacial growth in the postgenomic era. Semin Orthod. 2005;11:172–83.
8. Moss M, Salentijin L. The capsular matrix. Am J Orthod. 1969;56:474–90.
9. Moss M. The functional matrix hypothesis revisited. 1. The role of mechanotransduction. Am J Orthod Dentofacial Orthop. 1997a;112:8–11.
10. Moss M. The functional matrix hypothesis revisited. 2. The role of an osseous connected cellular network. Am J Orthod Dentofacial Orthop. 1997b;112:221–6.
11. Moss M. The functional matrix hypothesis revisited. 3. The genomic thesis. Am J Orthod Dentofacial Orthop. 1997c;112:338–42.
12. Moss M. The functional matrix hypothesis revisited. 4. The epigenetic antithesis and the resolving synthesis. Am J Orthod Dentofacial Orthop. 1997d;112:410–7.
13. Petrovic A. Postnatal growth of bone: a perspective of current trends, new approaches, and innovations. Prog Clin Biol Res. 1982;101:297–331.
14. Stutzmann J, Petrovic A. Role of the lateral pterygoid muscle and meniscotemporomandibular frenum in spontaneous growth of the mandible and in growth stimulated by the postural hyperpropulsor. Am J Orthod Dentofacial Orthop. 1990;97:381–92.
15. Lipton B. The biology of belief. Carlsbad, CA: Hay House, Inc.; 2008.
16. Dusheck J. It's the ecology, stupid! Nature. 2002;418:578–9.
17. Powell K. Stem-cell niches: it's the ecology, stupid! Nature. 2005;435:268–70.
18. Greene R, Pisano M. Palate morphogenesis: Current understanding and future directions. Birth Defects Res C Embryo Today. 2010;90:133–54.

19. Lipton B, Bensch K, Karasek M. Microvessel endothelial cell transdifferentiation: phenotypic characterization. Differentiation. 1991;46:117–33.
20. Lipton B, Bensch K, Karasek M. Histamine-modulated transdifferentiation of dermal microvascular endothelial cells. Exp Cell Res. 1992;199:279–91.
21. Netherwood T, Martin-Orue SM, O'Donnell AG, Gockling S, Graham J, GMathers JC, Gilbert HJ. Assessing the survival of transgenic plant DNA in the human gastrointestinal tract. Nat Biotechnol. 2004;22:204–9.
22. Steele E, Blanden R. Lamarck and antibody genes. Science. 2000;288:2318d–9d.
23. Nijhout H. The control of growth. Development. 2003;130:5863–7.
24. Center GSL. Epigenetics [Online]. University of Utah. 2008. http://learn.genetics.utah.edu/content/epigenetics/.
25. Willett W, Koplan J, Nugent R, Dusenbury C, Puska P, Gaziano T. Prevention of chronic disease by means of diet and lifestyle changes. Washington, DC: World Bank; 2006.
26. Chow K, Factor R, Ullman K. The nuclear envelope environment and its cancer connections. Nat Rev Cancer. 2012;12:196–209.
27. McGuinn L, Ghazarian A, Ellison G, Harvey C, Kaefer C, Reid B. Cancer and environment: definitions and misconceptions. Environ Res. 2012;112:230–4.
28. Peedicayil J. The role of DNA methylation in the pathogenesis and treatment of cancer. Curr Clin Pharmacol. 2012;7:333–40.
29. Gomes C, Trezza E, Murade E, Padovani C. Surface electromyography of facial muscles during natural and artificial feeding of infants. J Pediatr (Rio J). 2006;82:103–9.
30. Ovsenik M. Incorrect orofacial functions until 5 years of age and their association with posterior crossbite. Am J Orthod Dentofacial Orthop. 2009;136:375–81.
31. Lavergne J, Petrovic A. Discontinuities in occlusal relationship and the regulation of facial growth. A cybernetic view. Eur J Orthod. 1983;5:269–78.
32. Garn S, Cole P, Bailey S. Living together as a factor in family-line resemblances. Hum Biol. 1979;51:565–87.
33. De Muelenaere J, Wiltshire WA, Viljoen WP. The occlusal status of an urban and a rural Venda group. J Dent Assoc S Afr. 1992;47:517–20.
34. Otuyemi O, Abidoye R. Malocclusion in 12-year-old suburban and rural Nigerian children. Community Dent Health. 1993;10:375–80.
35. Von Cramon-Taubadel N. Global human mandibular variation reflects differences in agricultural and hunter-gatherer subsistence strategies. Proc Natl Acad Sci U S A. 2011;108:19546–51.
36. Du X, Hagg U. Muscular adaptation to gradual advancement of the mandible. Angle Orthod. 2003;73:525–31.
37. Grünheid T, Langenbach G, Korfage J, Zentner A, Van Eijden T. The adaptive response of jaw muscles to varying functional demands. Eur J Orthod. 2009;31:596–612.
38. Kiliaridis S, Mills C, Antonarakis G. Masseter muscle thickness as a predictive variable in treatment outcome of the twin-block appliance and masseteric thickness changes during treatment. Orthod Craniofac Res. 2010;13:203–13.
39. Liu Y, Behrents R, Buschang P. Mandibular growth, remodeling, and maturation during infancy and early childhood. Angle Orthod. 2010;80:97–105.
40. Miles T. Mastication, swallowing. In: Miles T, Nauntofte B, Svensson P, editors. Clinical oral physiology. Copenhagen: Quintessence Publishing Co. Ltd; 2004.
41. Nanda S. The developmental basis of occlusion and malocclusion. Chicago, IL: Quintessence Publishing Co. Ltd; 1983.
42. Frost H. A 2003 update of bone physiology and Wolff's law for clinicians. Angle Orthod. 2004;74:3–15.
43. Schoenau E, Frost H. The "muscle-bone unit" in children and adolescents. Calcif Tissue Int. 2002;70:405–7.
44. Gomes AC, Vitti M, Regalo S, Semprini M, Siessere S, Watanabe P, Palomari E. Evidence of muscle role over the cranio-facial skull development in Angle's Class III dental malocclusion under the clinical rest position. Electromyogr Clin Neurophysiol. 2008;48:335–41.

45. Colson S, Meekb J, Hawdonb J. Optimal positions for the release of primitive neonatal reflexes stimulating breastfeeding. Early Hum Dev. 2008;84:441–9.
46. López Del Valle L, Singh G, Feliciano N, Machuca MC. Associations between a history of breast feeding, malocclusion and parafunctional habits in Puerto Rican children. P R Health Sci J. 2006;25:31–4.
47. Menezes Kobayashi H, Scavone H Jr, Ferreira R, Gamba Garibb D. Relationship between breastfeeding duration and prevalence of posterior crossbite in the deciduous dentition. Am J Orthod Dentofacial Orthop. 2010;137:54–8.
48. Crelin E. The human vocal tract: anatomy, function, development, and evolution. New York, NY: Vantage Press; 1987.
49. Bosma J. Postnatal ontogeny of performances of the pharynx, larynx, and mouth. Am Rev Respir Dis. 1985;131:S10–5.
50. Fucile S, McFarland D, Gisel EG, Lau C. Oral and nonoral sensorimotor interventions facilitate suck-swallow-respiration functions and their coordination in preterm infants. Early Hum Dev. 2012;88:345–50.
51. Qureshi M, Vice F, Taciak V, Bosma J, Gewolb I. Changes in rhythmic suckle feeding patterns in term infants in the first month of life. Dev Med Child Neurol. 2002;44:34–9.
52. Gross A, Kellum G, Michas C, Franz D, Foster M, Walker M, Bishop F. Open-mouth posture and maxillary arch width in young children: a three-year evaluation. Am J Orthod Dentofacial Orthod. 1994;106:635–40.
53. Harari D, Redlich M, Miri S, Hamud T, Gross M. The effect of mouth breathing versus nasal breathing on dentofacial and craniofacial development in orthodontic patients. Laryngoscope. 2010;120:2089–93.
54. Serter S, Gunhan K, Can F, Pabuscu Y. Transformation of the maxillary bone in adults with nasal polyposis: a CT morphometric study. Diagn Interv Radiol. 2010;16:122–4.
55. Yamada T, Tanne K, Miyamoto K, Yamauchi K. Influences of nasal respiratory obstruction on craniofacial growth in young Macaca fuscata monkeys. Am J Orthod Dentofacial Orthop. 1997;111:38–43.
56. Aznar T, Galan A, Marin I, Dominguez A. Dental arch diameters and relationships to oral habits. Angle Orthod. 2006;76:441–5.
57. Page D. "Real" early orthodontic treatment. From birth to age 8. Funct Orthod. 2003;20:48–54.
58. Bishara S, Jakobsen J, Treder J, Nowak A. Arch width changes from 6 weeks to 45 years of age. Am J Orthod Dentofacial Orthop. 1997;111:401–9.
59. Van Der Linden FP. Facial growth and facial orthopedics. Chicago, IL: Quintessence Pub. Co; 1986.
60. Koenig J, Davies A, Thach B. Coordination of breathing, sucking, and swallowing during bottle feedings in human infants. J Appl Physiol. 1990;69:1623–9.
61. Sasaki C, Levine P, Laitman J, Crelin EJ. Postnatal descent of the epiglottis in man. A preliminary report. Arch Otolaryngol. 1977;103:169–71.
62. Tonkin S, Partridge J, Beach D, Whiteney S. The pharyngeal effect of partial nasal obstruction. Pediatrics. 1979;63:261–71.
63. Nowak A, Smith W, Erenberg A. Imaging evaluation of artificial nipples during bottle feeding. Arch Pediatr Adolesc Med. 1994;148:40–2.
64. Melink S, Vagner M, Hocevar-Boltezar I, Ovsenick M. Posterior crossbite in the deciduous dentition period, its relation with sucking habits, irregular orofacial functions, and otolaryngological findings. Am J Orthod Dentofacial Orthop. 2010;138:32–40.
65. Sánchez-Molins M, Grau Carbo J, Lischeid Gaig C, Ustrell Torrent J. Comparative study of the craniofacial growth depending on the type of lactation received. Eur J Paediatr Dent. 2010;11:87–92.
66. Carrascoza K, Possobon RDF, Tomita L, Moraes A. Consequences of bottle-feeding to the oral facial development of initially breastfed children. J Pediatr (Rio J). 2006;82:395–7.
67. Trawitzki L, Anselmo-Lima W, Melchior M, Grechi T, Valera F. Breast-feeding and deleterious oral habits in mouth and nose breathers. Braz J Otorhinolaryngol. 2005;71:747–51.

68. Viggiano D, Fasano D, Monaco G, Strohmenger L. Breast feeding, bottle feeding, and non-nutritive sucking; effects on occlusion in deciduous dentition. Arch Dis Child. 2004;89:1121–3.
69. Inoue N, Sakashitab R, Kamegal T. Reduction of masseter muscle activity in bottle-fed babies. Early Hum Dev. 1995;42:185–93.
70. Neiva F, Wertzner H. A protocol for oral myofunctional assessment: for application with children. Int J Orofacial Myology. 1996;22:8–19.
71. Simoes W. Insights into maxillary and mandibular growth for a better practice. J Clin Pediatr Dent. 1996;21:1–8.
72. Ramirez-Yañez G. Early treatment of malocclusions Cucuta. Cúcuta: J Ramirez Press; 2009.
73. Liu Z, Ikeda K, Harada S, Kasahara Y, Ito G. Functional properties of jaw and tongue muscles in rats fed a liquid diet after being weaned. J Dent Res. 1998;77:366–76.
74. Ravosa M, Ning J, Costley D, Daniel A, Stock S, Stack M. Masticatory biomechanics and masseter fiber-type plasticity. J Musculoskelet Neuronal Interact. 2010;10:46–55.
75. James G, Strokon D. Cranial strains and malocclusion VII: a review. Int J Orthod Milwaukee. 2006;17:23–8.
76. Ng A, Yang Y, Wong R, Hagg E, Rabie A. Factors regulating condylar cartilage growth under repeated load application. Front Biosci. 2006;11:949–54.
77. Alaqeel S, Hinton R, Opperman L. Cellular response to force application at craniofacial sutures. Orthod Craniofac Res. 2006;9:111–22.
78. Opperman L, Rawlins J. The extracellular matrix environment in suture morphogenesis and growth. Cells Tissues Organs. 2005;181:127–35.
79. Ramirez-Yañez G, Daley T, Symons A, Young W. Incisor disocclusion in rats affects mandibular condylar cartilage at the cellular level. Arch Oral Biol. 2004a;49:393–400.
80. Smartt J, Low D, Barlett S. The pediatric mandible: I. A primer on growth and development. Plast Reconstr Surg. 2005;116:14e–23e.
81. Sillman J. Serial study of good occlusion from birth to 12 years of age. Am J Orthod. 1951;37:481–507.
82. Westover K, Diloreto M, Shearer T. The relationship of breastfeeding to oral development and dental concerns. ASDC J Dent Child. 1989;56:140–3.
83. Stuart-Macadam P, Dettwyler K. Breastfeeding: biocultural perspectives. Piscataway, NJ: Transaction Publishers; 1995.
84. Mølgaard C, Larnkjaer A, Mark A Michaelsen K. Are early growth and nutrition related to bone health in adolescence? The Copenhagen Cohort Study of infant nutrition and growth. Am J Clin Nutr. 2011;94:1865S–9S.
85. Gomes C, Thomson Z, Cardoso J. Utilization of surface electromyography during the feeding of term and preterm infants: a literature review. Dev Med Child Neurol. 2009;51:936–42.
86. Gungor A, Turkkahraman H. Effects of airway problems on maxillary growth: a review. Eur J Dent. 2009;3:250–4.
87. Fielding J, Gilchick R. Positioning for prevention from day 1 (and before). Breastfeed Med. 2011;6:249–55.
88. Hauck F, Thompson J, Tanabe K, Moon R, Vennemann M. Breastfeeding and reduced risk of sudden infant death syndrome: a meta-analysis. Pediatrics. 2011;128:103–10.
89. Zotter H, Pichler G. Breast feeding is associated with decreased risk of sudden infant death syndrome. Evid Based Med. 2012;17:126–7.
90. Corruccini R. An epidemiologic transition in dental occlusion in world populations. Am J Orthod. 1984;86:419–26.
91. Corruccini R. How anthropology informs the orthodontic diagnosis of malocclusion's causes. Lewiston, NY: Teh Edwin Mellen Press; 1999.
92. Simoes W. Ortopedia Funcional de los Maxilares - vista a traves de la rehabilitacion neuro-oclusal. São Paulo: Artes Medicas; 2003.
93. Vargervik K, Miller A, Chierici G, Harvold E, Tomer B. Morphologic response to changes in neuromuscular patterns experimentally induced by altered modes of respiration. Am J Orthod. 1984;85:115–24.

94. Cuccia A, Lotti M, Caradonna D. Oral breathing and head posture. Angle Orthod. 2008;78:77–82.
95. Miller A, Vargervik K, Chierici G. Sequential neuromuscular changes in rhesus monkeys during the initial adaptation to oral respiration. Am J Orthod. 1982;81:99–107.
96. Rodenstein D, Stǎnescu D. Soft palate and oronasal breathing in humans. J Appl Physiol. 1984;57:651–7.
97. Kayukawa H. Malocclusion and masticatory muscle activity: a comparison of four types of malocclusion. J Clin Pediatr Dent. 1992;16:162–77.
98. Kiliaridis S, Mejersjo C, Thilander B. Muscle function and craniofacial morphology: a clinical study in patients with myotonic dystrophy. Eur J Orthod. 1989;11:131–8.
99. Lear C, Moorrees C. Buccolingual muscle force and dental arch form. Am J Orthod. 1969;56:379–93.
100. De Freitas M, Alcazar N, Janson G, De Freitas K, Henriques J. Upper and lower pharyngeal airways in subjects with Class I and Class II malocclusions and different growth patterns. Am J Orthod Dentofacial Orthop. 2006;130:742–5.
101. Moore K, Dalley A, Agur A. Clinically oriented anatomy. 6th ed. Baltimore, MD: Lippincott Williams & Wilkins; 2010.
102. Marks M. Recognizing the allergic person. Am Fam Physician. 1977;16:72–9.
103. Oliveira A, Dos Anjos C, Silva E, Menezes PDL. Indicative factors of early facial aging in mouth breathing adults. Pro Fono. 2007;19:305–12.
104. Freeman K, Bonuck K. Snoring, mouth-breathing, and apnea trajectories in a population-based cohort followed from infancy to 81 months: a cluster analysis. Int J Pediatr Otorhinolaryngol. 2012;76:122–30.
105. Izu S, Itamoto C, Pradella-Hallinan M, Pizarro G, Tufik S, Pignatari S, Fujita R. Obstructive sleep apnea syndrome (OSAS) in mouth breathing children. Braz J Otorhinolaryngol. 2010;76:552–6.
106. Carra M, Huynh N, Morton P, Rompre P, Papadakis A, Remise C, Lavigne G. Prevalence and risk factors of sleep bruxism and wake-time tooth clenching in a 7- to 17-yr-old population. Eur J Oral Sci. 2011;119:386–94.
107. Spahis J. Sleepless nights: obstructive sleep apnea in the pediatric patient. Pediatr Nurs. 1994;20:469–72.
108. Ramirez-Yañez G, Smid J, Young W, Waters M. Influence of growth hormone on the craniofacial complex of transgenic mice. Eur J Orthod. 2005;27:494–500.
109. Ramirez-Yañez G, Young W, Daley T, Waters M. Influence of growth hormone on the mandibular condylar cartilage of rats. Arch Oral Biol. 2004b;49:585–90.
110. Velloso C. Regulation of muscle mass by growth hormone and IGF-I. Br J Pharmacol. 2008;154:557–68.
111. Young W, Ramirez-Yañez G, Daley T, Smid J, Coshigano K, Kopchick J, Waters M. Growth hormone and epidermal growth factor in salivary glands of giant and dwarf transgenic mice. J Histochem Cytochem. 2004;52:1191–7.
112. Nowak A, Warren J. Infant oral health and oral habits. Pediatr Clin North Am. 2000;47:1043–66.
113. Moses A. Thumb sucking or thumb propping? CDS Rev. 1987;80:40–2.
114. Thüer U, Sieber R, Ingerval B. Cheek and tongue pressures in the molar areas and the atmospheric pressure in the palatal vault in young adults. Eur J Orthod. 1999;21:299–309.
115. Görgülü S, Sagdic D, Akin E, Karacay S, Bulakbasi N. Tongue movements in patients with skeletal Class III malocclusions evaluated with real-time balanced turbo field echo cine magnetic resonance imaging. Am J Orthod Dentofacial Orthop. 2011;139:e405–14.
116. Primozic J, Farcnik F, Perinetti G, Richmond S, Ovsenik M. The association of tongue posture with the dentoalveolar maxillary and mandibular morphology in Class III malocclusion: a controlled study. Eur J Orthod. 2012;35:388–93.
117. Yılmaz F, Sagdic D, Karacay S, Akin E, Bulakbasi N. Tongue movements in patients with skeletal Class II malocclusion evaluated with real-time balanced turbo field echo cine magnetic resonance imaging. Am J Orthod Dentofacial Orthop. 2011;139:e415–25.

118. Baccetti T, Franchi L, McNamara JJ, Tollaro I. Early dentofacial features of Class II malocclusion: a longitudinal study from the deciduous through the mixed dentition. Am J Orthod Dentofacial Orthop. 1997;111:502–9.
119. Lux C, Burden D, Conradt C, Komposch G. Age-related changes in sagittal relationship between the maxilla and mandible. Eur J Orthod. 2005;27:568–78.
120. Stahl F, Baccetti T, Franchi L, McNamara JAJR. Longitudinal growth changes in untreated subjects with Class II Division 1 malocclusion. Am J Orthod Dentofacial Orthop. 2008;134:125–37.
121. Musich D, Busch M. Early orthodontic treatment: current clinical perspectives. Alpha Omegan. 2007;100:17–24.
122. Ackerman J, Proffit W. Soft tissue limitations in orthodontics: treatment planning guidelines. Angle Orthod. 1997;67:327–36.
123. Ramirez-Yañez G, Farrell C. Soft tissue dysfunction: a missing clue when treating malocclusions. Int J Jaw Funct Orthoped. 2005;1:351–9.
124. Smithpeter J, Covell DJ. Relapse of anterior open bites treated with orthodontic appliances with and without orofacial myofunctional therapy. Am J Orthod Dentofacial Orthop. 2010;137:605–14.
125. Thilander B, Rubio G, Pena L, De Mayorga C. Prevalence of temporomandibular dysfunction and its association with malocclusion in children and adolescents: an epidemiologic study related to specified stages of dental development. Angle Orthod. 2002;72:146–54.
126. Guillminault C, Akhtar F. Pediatric sleep-disordered breathing: New evidence on its development. Sleep Med Rev. 2015;24:46–56.
127. Huang Y, Guilleminault C. Pediatric obstructive sleep apnea and the critical role of oral-facial growth: evidences. Front Neurol. 2013;3:1–7.

Craniofacial Signs, Symptoms and Orthodontic Objectives of Paediatric Obstructive Sleep Apnoea

4

Seng-Mun (Simon) Wong

4.1   Introduction

The study of craniofacial growth and development has a long history in the disciplines of Paediatric Dentistry and Orthodontics. Unbalanced facial growth is known to be causative for dental misalignment and malocclusion. However, historically, little emphasis has been placed on the possible link to obstructive sleep apnoea. Through greater understanding from contemporary studies and reflections from past research, we now are bringing to light the interrelationships of all proximal structures in the many chronic issues that ail our children.

When studied with the context to link the maxillomandibular complex with pharyngeal patency and sleep breathing disorders, many signs and symptoms are present. When care is taken to evaluate the facial structures of the growing child, clear indicators of development issues and their connection with airway dysfunction are observable.

Clues from definitive corrective treatments for obstructive sleep apnoea may give us reason to consider changes in orthodontic operative standards. Treatment objectives accounting for the orthodontic impact on the airway will hopefully expand future markers for success to encompass improving balance for the whole craniofacial complex.

S.-M. (Simon). Wong (✉)
Private Practice, Melbourne, VIC, Australia

Orthotropics Module, Department of Orthodontics, University of Valencia, Valencia, Spain

© Springer Nature Switzerland AG 2019   57
E. Liem (ed.), *Sleep Disorders in Pediatric Dentistry*,
https://doi.org/10.1007/978-3-030-13269-9_4

4.2   Orthodontic Context for Obstructive Sleep Apnoea

Obstructive sleep apnoea (OSA) is a dysfunction during sleep characterized by recurrent, episodic cessation of breath due to complete or partial blockage of the upper airway. It is a high-order part of a spectrum of upper airway dysfunctions within the sleep disorder breathing syndromes (SDBS).

Although all the related disorders within the spectrum of SDBS are diagnosed and managed by medical practitioners, Kaditis et al. [1] as part of the European Respiratory Society Task Force now recommends adjunctive orthognathics and orthodontics be included in stepwise care for SDBS.

Orthodontic observations provide vital clues to airway performance. Misaligned teeth and distorted jaws are but hard tissue evidence of craniofacial aberrations of the structures associated with upper airway obstructions. Huang and Guilleminault [2] overviewed this and reflected many decades of linking disorders of oral-facial growth and OSA in children.

To understand the association of malocclusion and OSA, it is useful to review how malocclusion develops. Specifically, Dibbets [3] indicated the maxilla set too far down or back or too small in form is the genesis of malocclusion. Björk [4] measured ideal maxillary growth at a mean of 51 degrees and later Ruf et al. [5] mandibular growth at 54 degrees. Both noted good overall alignment with these growth directions but considerable variations of increased vertical growth associated with malocclusions. McNamara [6] highlighted that even in Angle's Class II malocclusions most commonly the maxilla was retrusive and excess height of the lower face the most common finding.

Platou and Zachrisson [7] then confirmed patients with more horizontal growth tendencies of "prognathia" (forward jaws) had straighter teeth and better balance in facial form than vertical growing "retrognathia" (retruded jaws).

The most typical orthodontic cluster of findings in SDBS was illuminated by Linder-Aronson [8] many decades previously:

> The results have shown that children who had difficulties in nasal breathing were characterized by increases in both the lower and total facial heights, the sagittal depth of the bony nasopharynx was less, the tongue had a lower position, the upper arch was narrow, the upper and lower incisors were retroclined, the palatal vault was of normal height, there was a cross-bite or tendency towards cross-bite, a tendency towards open bite and normal antero-posterior relationship between upper and lower jaws. Disturbed nasal respiration can affect both facial morphology and the dentition.

Hultcrantz and Lofstrand [9] and Kim and Guilleminault [10] reconfirmed these findings in recent studies.

Craniofacial aberrations and distortions cannot but impact the function of its organs and efficiency of the body's actions. Less than optimal form and imbalances in structures of the soft and hard tissues of the face reduce all its potential. Developmental distress can present as dysfunction of mastication, communication and of course breathing.

There are two aperture areas with two segments in the upper respiratory pathways; two nostrils and the mouth lead, respectively, to the nasopharynx and the oropharynx.

Any reductions in maxilla size, distortions in its shape and/or incorrect location of its positioning can reduce nasopharyngeal airflow efficiency. Increase in soft tissue mass of the turbinates, the adenoids and the tonsils are also obstructive; however, Migueis et al. [11] concluded nasal and nasopharyngeal level issues, important in SDBS, play only a minor role in the more extreme disorder of OSA. Venkamp et al. [12] confirms this by also discarding the relevance of obstructions at or above the oropharyngeal level, voiding the relevance of the usual suspect set of adenoids and tonsils when dealing with OSA.

Of highest significance then are the hyoid level obstructions. Any loss of tone, overcrowding of the intraoral space and dysfunction in the glossus muscles (tongue) and the mandible elevator muscles result in the hanging of the mandible and resting with the mouth open. This postural weakness has the potential in the supine sleep position for further flexion of the head/neck that can collapse all the soft tissues interlinked with the hyoid bone and the posterior pharyngeal wall.

An open-mouth posture must be one of the key indicators to assess for as it is commonly intertwined with mouth breathing tendencies, which, by default, is already a laboured means of respiration. The genesis of this incorrect oral posture is likely from nasal and nasopharyngeal congestions and obstructions, though De Felicio et al. [13] suggests weakness and poor functional muscular coordination.

Surprisingly, though the signs and symptoms of poor oral posture are obvious to the eye, they are largely ignored. Glatz-Noll and Berg [14] discovered normal (the clinical control subjects) industrialized 4-year-olds on average leave their mouths open for 83.3% of the time, yet few even today appear to place any significance to these findings.

Trotman et al. [15] however elucidated a very powerful interrelationship with the soft and hard tissues of the maxillomandibular complex:

A more open lip posture was associated with a downward and backward rotation of the maxilla and mandible a more obtuse gonial angle, a retruded mandible with retroclined incisors, extruded maxillary molars and maxillary and mandibular incisors, and an elongated total face height caused mainly by a larger anterior face height.

To truly understand the dental/facial/head/neck relationship to airway flow, the equilibrium balance of space management in the body organ relationship needs recognition. Each structure of the body requires a minimum volume with correct spatial placement to work effectively. Luzi [16] showed a consistency in biological form that adapted the base of skull saddle Ba S N angle and maxilla/mandible ANB angle relative relationships to very precise arrangements (Fig. 4.1).

Less than 2.5-degrees was found within the group of 160 Class I subjects measured indicating very tight volumetric requirements for the head and face.

The growing structures adapt to environmental change but must maintain overall spatial requirements for function. To some extent, form can change but not overall

Saddle Angle
SNA
115.5
89
Saddle Angle
SNA
140
64.5
115.5 + 89 = 204.5
140 + 64.5 = 204.5

Fig. 4.1 Luzi [16] showed a consistency in biological form that adapted the base of skull saddle Ba S N angle and maxilla/mandible ANB angle relative relationships to very precise arrangements

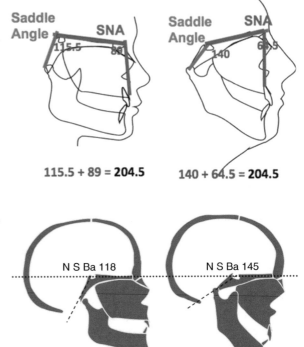

N S Ba 118
N S Ba 145

Fig. 4.2 Remodelling occurs in the vertical ramus forward, and a reduction in the horizontal ramus coincides to rebalance the angles necessary for the best equilibrium of the balance of all the structures

volume. In children who maintain an open-mouth posture, when the unsupported maxilla "drops," the mandible must change rotational position to maintain the excess freeway space adopted. This has an unwanted consequence of shifting the tongue at the hyoid level to close pharyngeal space. In order to protect the airway, the mandible in the growing child, in time, must change its form too.

Remodelling occurs in the vertical ramus forward, and a reduction in the horizontal ramus coincides to rebalance the angles necessary for the best equilibrium of the balance of all the structures (Fig. 4.2). In the growing child as enormous changes occur over short periods of time, the adaptations of bony structures to soft tissue-induced poor posture can be disproportionally large.

Trenouth and Timms [17] measured 20-degree difference in saddle angles between well-balanced faces with good dental alignment and distorted faces with dental misalignment.

In children with high saddle angle growth, in addition to the maxilla and mandible being down and back, the arch lengths are shorter and teeth crowded. As Bernabe et al. [18] confirmed arch length to be the deciding factor in dental crowding, it is clear the anterior-posterior dimensions are also critical for optimal placement of the tongue in the intraoral cavity.

Marcotte [19] and Vig [20] observed a further postural compensation occurs when the mouth is left open at rest. The cervical vertebra curves forward to allow the extension of the cranium on the atlas, so the weight of the head balances and the eyes level to the horizon. In compensation the head is tipped up for ease in breathing with the neck and shoulders rolled forward to allow the eyes to level for ambulatory balance.

In the airway-compromised, the head is routinely rotated to keep nasion forehead/nose juncture above pogonian of the lower jaw chin.

4.3   The Facial Clues

With these considerations, there are many signs and symptoms revealing of structural and functional problems in the growing child's face and mouth. Mew [21] outlines oral and head postural problems that highlight childhood development issues.

A sloping forehead can foretell of imbalances, as likely head tilt compensation is present (Fig. 4.3). Typically in compromised postures, the forehead is tilted back or down, both placing the head in a forward position. A forehead when in the upright stance should be roughly perpendicular to level ground and in line with the chest. When the head is reset to this level, a truer relative position of the facial jaws in their horizontal and vertical growth direction can be shown (Fig. 4.4).

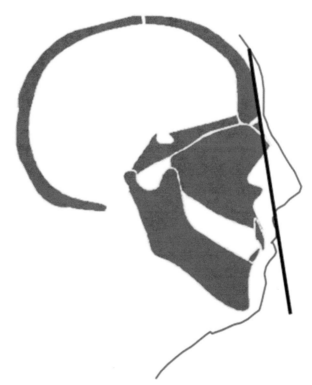

Fig. 4.3 A sloping forehead can foretell of imbalances, as likely head tilt compensation is present

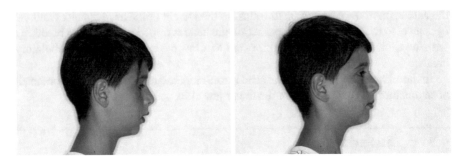

Fig. 4.4 When the head is reset to this level, a truer relative position of the facial jaws in their horizontal and vertical growth direction can be shown

The cheek line

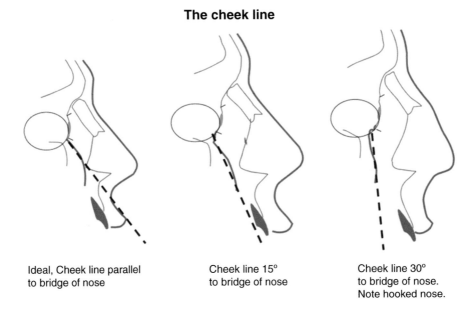

Ideal, Cheek line parallel to bridge of nose

Cheek line 15° to bridge of nose

Cheek line 30° to bridge of nose. Note hooked nose.

Fig. 4.5 In good balanced faces, the cheek line runs parallel with the nasal bones

A correctly placed maxilla in an up and forward position tends to carry the nose tip up in line with the stably positioned nasal bones. Straight noses have good nasal and maxilla bone support. Correctly placed and sized maxilla offers significant support in the soft tissue structures around the eyes and strongly defines the cheekbones. In good balanced faces, the cheek line runs parallel with the nasal bones (Fig. 4.5).

A break in the nose line can be very revealing of much deeper changes in the facial bone complex. Facial bone development that is in a back and downward direction results in flattening of the zygomatic cheekbone lines and drop away from the line of the nasal bones. Cheekbones present as soft and flat, and the soft tissue

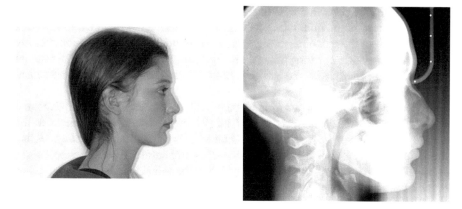

Fig. 4.6 A hooknose or angle change from the nasal bone inclination to nose tip tells of less forward and more vertical growth

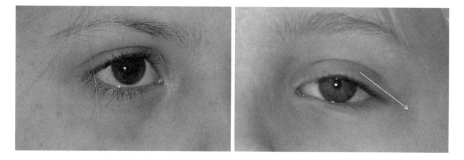

Fig. 4.7 Even the eyelid levels are impacted by the growth trend direction of the maxilla

form of the face including the tip of the nose is drawn down away from the line of the nasal bones.

A hooknose or angle change from the nasal bone inclination to nose tip tells of less forward and more vertical growth (Fig. 4.6).

Even the eyelid levels are impacted by the growth trend direction of the maxilla (Fig. 4.7). Well-positioned maxillae offer good support of the soft tissues overlaying them, so they uplift the eyelids and no whites under the iris should show. When white sclera is noticeably visible under the irises and downward turn of the canthus (outer corner) of eyelid appears as a sleepy droop, then underlying cheekbone fullness is lacking, and there is good indication of the lack of forward projection of the maxilla in growth.

Further down the face, more soft tissue markers tell of muscle tone weakness or dysfunction. Cheek muscle bulge or hollowness is very revealing of levels of muscle tone. Ongoing overuse of the buccinator muscles indicates lack of maturity in the swallow pattern. Incorrect muscle function influences growth in the immature bones of young children as it impacts both functional action and resting posture.

Facial muscles (buccinator, orbicularis oris, mentalis) and the tongue driving forward are used in the infant for suckling. This is normally scheduled to shift to a predominance of the mandible elevator muscles (temporalis, masseter) for chewing and the tongue gently uplifting for swallowing in the second year of life. This should coincide with eruption of the primary molar teeth and the time of anatomical readiness for speech.

In correct development, suckling changes fully to swallowing, but Matsuo and Palmer [22] and Van De Engel-Hoek et al. [23] note various disturbances to the natural cycle of neuromuscular coordination as being commonplace today. Unlike the quiet nature of the mature swallow, this compensatory hybrid type "suck-swallow" is excessively busy because much like the infant suckles, all the muscles of the mouth and face appear to fire simultaneously. Machado et al. [24] and Almiro et al. [25] revealed radiologically how these parafunctions are detrimental to airway patency in the dentate child.

Visually this presents as over-retention of "baby cheeks" and excessive lower lip activity and chin "dimpling" due to disruptions of the learning process needed to quieten the face in adult deglutition (Fig. 4.8).

Brace [26] hypothesised one possible culprit for this phenomenon: spoon-feeding infants who are only capable of suckling liquids, before their time for neurobiological development of lip seal swallow for solids.

Correct lip form is dual symmetric, even in tone in both upper and lower jaw and without eversion past the dry/wet line of the inner oral surfaces. Asymmetry in lip form is observable when developmental control is poor (Fig. 4.9). Lip unevenness with tight thinner upper lip, everted, flaccid, overly full lower lip and downturned corner commissures signify improper muscle tone and control.

Good habitual lip together resting from toned temporalis and masseter elevator muscles presents a natural tendency to leave the lips softly together in the resting posture. In poor function lip seal is only fleetingly present, often without touching during in speech and, when in contact, "purse forced" under tension (Fig. 4.10).

It is important also to be observant for facial (and general body) signs of obesity, which Mathew and Narang [27] note has a 50% association with childhood apnoea. Being overweight is neither a normal nor healthy characteristic. Narang and Mathew [28] states in children with OSA "obesity may independently or synergistically magnify the underlying cardiovascular and metabolic burden".

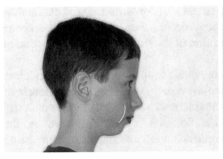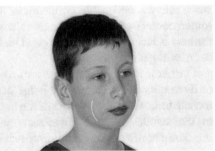

Fig. 4.8 Visually this presents as over-retention of "baby cheeks"

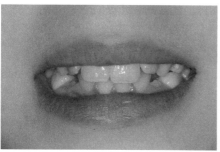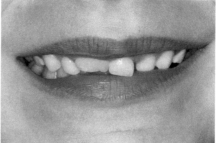

Fig. 4.9   Asymmetry in lip form is observable when developmental control is poor

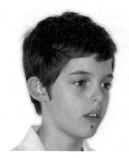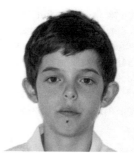

Fig. 4.10   In poor function lip seal is only fleetingly present, often without touching during in speech and when in contact, "purse forced" under tension

Incidentally but equally pertinent, parallel signs of excessive decay are commonly found in these children. Unsurprisingly, Ruanpeng et al. [29] recognises the culprit for much of their problems as the age-old dental nemesis, excess sugar consumption.

4.4   Orthodontic Clues

Skeletal and dental assessments standard to orthodontic evaluations for malocclusion can be very useful when searching for insights into compromised airways. Flores-Mir et al. [30] points out key associations with retrusive chin, steep mandibular plane, vertical direction of growth and a tendency towards Class II malocclusion and OSA. Reviewing the child, in for routine orthodontic evaluations, with an airway centric mindset can be advantageous for the health-compromised child.

Normally malocclusion misalignment of the jaws and teeth is categorised by their vertical and horizontal relationships using the Angle's classification of malocclusion.

Class I Crowding: Upper and lower jaws in even balance. Crowding or spacing misalignments limited to teeth. Good muscle tone in general. There will still be some reduction in tongue space as growth forward is still reduced from ideal, if there is insufficient arch length for all 32 permanent teeth. Posturally, lip seal is good at rest, but teeth are left slightly apart and tongue is off the palate in the posterior 1/3 and likely resting between the molars (Fig. 4.11).

Class II Division 1: Lower jaw behind upper. Size and form distortions notable with weakened muscle tone. Both jaws are back with the lower weaker of the two. Crowding of the teeth is minimal but the upper incisors are proclined forward. Tongue is completely off the palate, laying on the lower teeth at rest and at hyoid level further back in pharyngeal throat space. The mouth is open at rest with jaw swung back with a large freeway space, as overall tone is poor (Fig. 4.12).

Class II Division 2: Both jaws set back with lower cupped up within upper. Jaw length is shortened and crowding of teeth found both at front and back of arch. Distortions are found in shape and form from strong but uncontrolled muscle tone. Upper front teeth are retroclined. Joints are often compressed back and tongue space tight with spreading out broadly between molar teeth so dental misalignments are usually noticeable. Lips are tightly sealed at rest, but teeth are always apart (Fig. 4.13).

Class III Low Angle: Lower jaw ahead of upper jaw, with upper smaller by a degree. Space is tight for upper teeth, but good alignment is found in the lower arch though in both arches the incisors are retroclined. Tongue space is good in the lower arch but insufficient in the upper so the maxilla is unsupported and growth has a

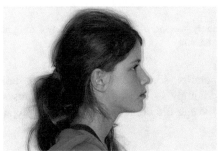
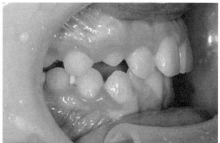

Fig. 4.11 Class I crowding

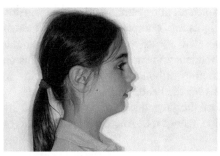
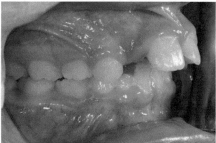

Fig. 4.12 Class II division 1

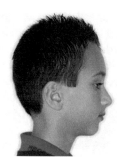

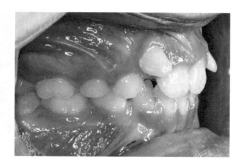

Fig. 4.13 Class II division 2

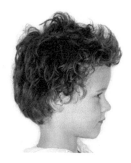

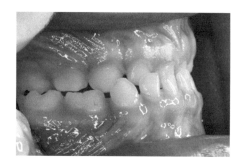

Fig. 4.14 Class III low angle

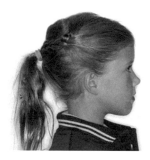

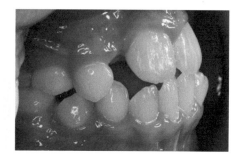

Fig. 4.15 Class III high angle

hidden vertical tendency. Lowered tongue posture is kept in mouth often due to obstructions further back from enlarged tonsils or just a habit of resting low. Good muscle tone but mouth open and lower jaw held forward at rest (Fig. 4.14).

Class III High Angle: Lower jaw ahead of upper with divergent growth directions. Tongue space is rarely adequate in either arch. Nasal and throat obstructions from adenoids and tonsils are common. Sleep breathing disorder symptoms are common. Mouth is open at rest and tongue held down firmly (Fig. 4.15).

Excess Vertical Growth: Jaws divergent with long face presentation with both jaws down and back. Significant distortions in form and crowding are common.

Tongue held between all teeth at rest. Intraoral tongue space is deficient and airways compromised in multiple levels along the pharyngeal space. SBD symptoms abound. Weak muscle tone. Mouth mostly open and jaw down and back (Fig. 4.16).

Open Bite: Teeth not meeting at the front are characteristic of incomplete bites where the tongue rests forward and the mouth is kept open. Tongue space is compromised in throat and mouth and appears proportionately large and very strong. Often with functional non nutritive suckling habits. Mouth always open with tongue held forward past teeth (Fig. 4.17).

The soft tissue organs and boundaries of the mouth are important to consider when gauging airway patency. Looking into the open mouth can be most revealing. Mallampati (Fig. 4.18) scoring is a diagnostic tool used by anaesthetists to reveal the level of "congestion" within the mouth, blocking their access to the throat space.

When reviewing for potential airway issues, the tongue to available intraoral space relationship in the mouth is the most easily observable of the many signs. Without sufficient intraoral space in the closed bite resting position for the tongue, the tongue will either have to back off into the throat or come forward out past the lips. Ubiquitous to this forward tongue resting children is nasal congestion and mouth breathing tendency (Fig. 4.19).

The glossus muscle is the central organ of the mouth. It occupies an enormous percentage of the oral cavity, and it is concurrently the front boundary of the pharyngeal throat space. A tongue tight for intraoral space or just habitually resting

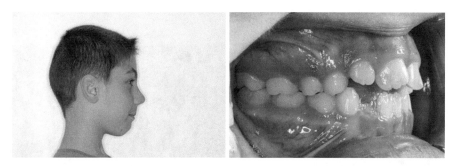

Fig. 4.16 Excess vertical growth

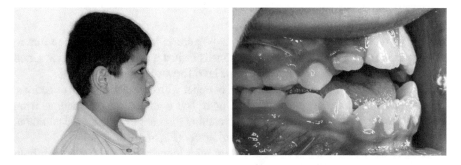

Fig. 4.17 Open bite

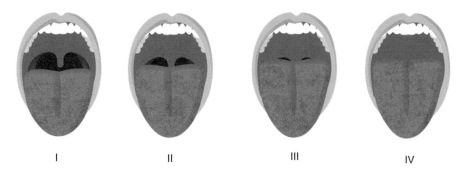

I   II   III   IV

Fig. 4.18 Mallampati scoring

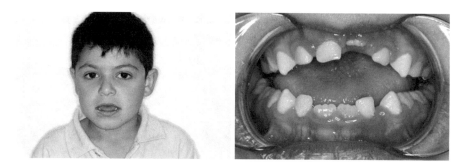

Fig. 4.19 Ubiquitous to this forward tongue resting children is nasal congestion and mouth breathing tendency

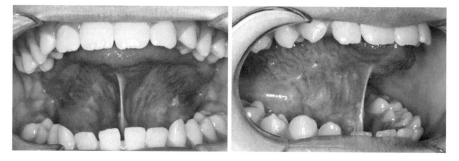

Fig. 4.20 Untreated short lingual frenulum

back will impact throat space volume in the oropharynx and the pharynx at the hyoid bone level.

Outside of the obviousness of excessive tongue size, Guilleminault et al. [31] links untreated short lingual frenulum (Fig. 4.20) with obstructive sleep breathing syndrome at later age.

Ankyloglossia tongue-ties range from complete to mild depending on the proximity of the tether to the tip (Fig. 4.21). The tether to the floor of mouth

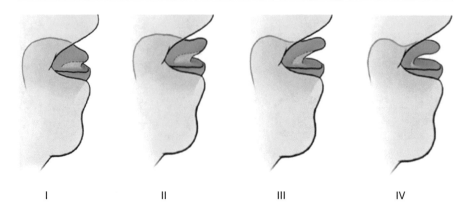

I   II   III   IV

Fig. 4.21 Ankyloglossia tongue-ties range from complete to mild depending on the proximity of the tether to the tip

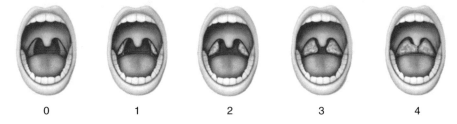

0   1   2   3   4

Fig. 4.22 Grading tonsils

normally should be more than 16 mm from the tip of the tongue, but many infants and children show reduced range of tongue mobility from being overbound to the mouth floor.

Further back, ear/nose/throat surgeons grade tonsil size for the purpose of evaluating their inflammation levels and potential for obstruction (Fig. 4.22). These tools all can be recruited for orthodontic use to check issues of the oropharynx.

Low-draped soft palate, flaccid, enlarged uvula and hypertrophic and inflamed tonsils take up valuable pharyngeal real estate (Fig. 4.23). It is unclear if mouth breathing and lowered tongue postures are the cause or the effect of the enlarged tonsils, but they should nonetheless be included in routine examinations.

Dental arch form provides much information when viewed with the airway in mind (Fig. 4.24). High and narrow palate with prominent rugae will usually indicate tongue in lower, retruded and disruptive position as rest. Tongues that are tight for space in the mouth rest either back, down, laterally or forward off the palate, often creating much disruption of the teeth alignment as well.

Crossbites are often found in children with OSA (Fig. 4.25). When the lower jaw or teeth arch form is broader or longer than in the upper, the lower crosses past the upper when biting. In all situations the tongue is displaced more posteriorly mouth and takes up valuable pharyngeal space.

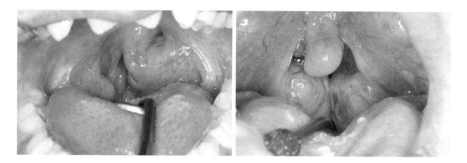

Fig. 4.23 Low-draped soft palate, flaccid, enlarged uvula, and hypertrophic and inflamed tonsils take up valuable pharyngeal real estate

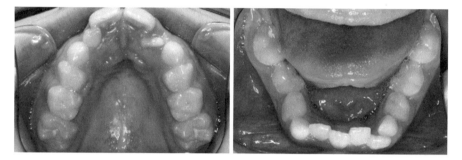

Fig. 4.24 Dental arch form provides much information when viewed with the airway in mind

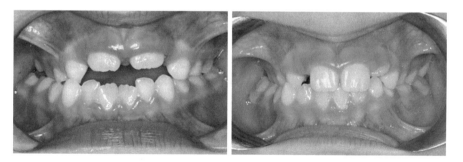

Fig. 4.25 Crossbites are often found in children with OSA

Mew [21] charts an in-depth relationship between the resting tongue and the intraoral arch dimensions at the palatal gingival margins of the upper first molars (Fig. 4.26). There is cause to believe the narrower the upper arch, the lower the tongue sits in the mouth.

Any widespread disease states found in the dentition can also be valuable clues. Enamel erosion and generalised decay may be symptomatic of gastroesophageal reflux common to OSA. Noronha et al. [32] and Ranjitkar et al. [33] record

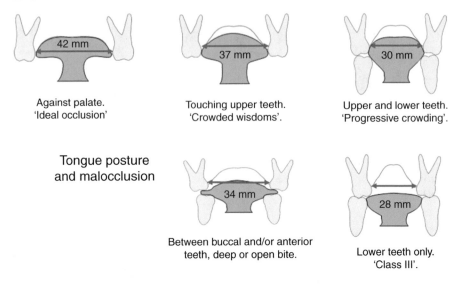

Against palate.
'Ideal occlusion'

Touching upper teeth.
'Crowded wisdoms'.

Upper and lower teeth.
'Progressive crowding'.

**Tongue posture
and malocclusion**

Between buccal and/or anterior
teeth, deep or open bite.

Lower teeth only.
'Class III'.

Fig. 4.26 Mew [21] charts an in-depth relationship between the resting tongue and the intraoral arch dimensions at the palatal gingival margins of the upper first molars

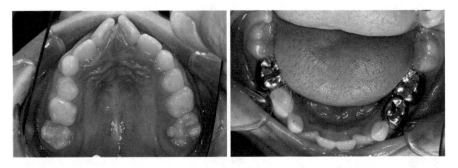

Fig. 4.27 Affected teeth will be either already restored with composite fillings or stainless steel crowns or extracted early

correlation and rising incidence in childhood OSA with dental damage caused by acid regurgitation.

Often the orthodontist will not see the eroded occlusal surfaces with "dished out" dentine exposure, but instead the initial presentation will be full-coverage restorations of the teeth throughout the mouth (Fig. 4.27). As the paediatric dentist will have already been primary carer for these children, affected teeth will be either already restored with composite fillings or stainless steel crowns or extracted early.

Standard X-ray used for all diagnostics in orthodontic care can also be used to show upper airway obstructions (Fig. 4.28). Major et al. [34] concluded soft tissue obstructions in the nasopharynx; the oropharynx is easily traceable and reasonably reliable for screening purposes. In addition Vieira et al. [35] correlated increased

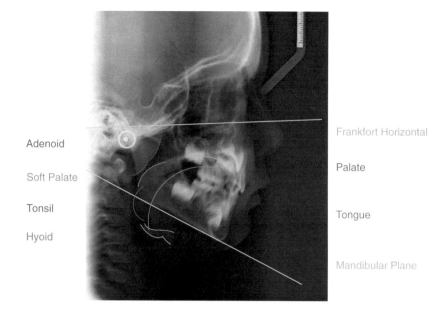

Adenoid

Soft Palate

Tonsil

Hyoid

Frankfort Horizontal

Palate

Tongue

Mandibular Plane

Fig. 4.28 Standard cephalometric X-ray

vertical facial height and anterior and inferior position of the hyoid bone to be predictive for obstructive sleep apnoea in children.

4.5 Malformation Syndromes

Unfortunately Kaditis et al. [1] reports OSA to be all too common a finding in syndromic malformations. Normally these syndromes are organised in four general categories of relevance for their medico-dental management teams:

- Mandibular deficiency: e.g. Pierre Robin, Stickler and Treacher Collins
- Mandibular prognathism: e.g. Marfan, Downs and Crouzon
- Facial height problems: e.g. amelogenesis imperfecta
- Facial asymmetry: e.g. hemifacial microsomia

Unquestionably, extreme distortions of the maxilla and mandible impact vital function from birth. Cleft lip and palate present as the most common issue with the maxilla (Fig. 4.29).

In the micrognathic extreme undersized mandible, there is always a threat to airway function, e.g. Pierre Robin syndrome (Fig. 4.30) and Stickler syndrome (Fig. 4.31).

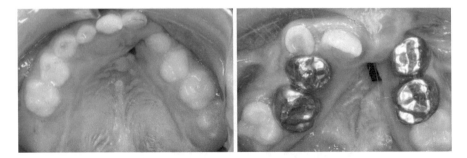

Fig. 4.29 Cleft lip and palate present as the most common issue with the maxilla

Fig. 4.30 Pierre Robin syndrome

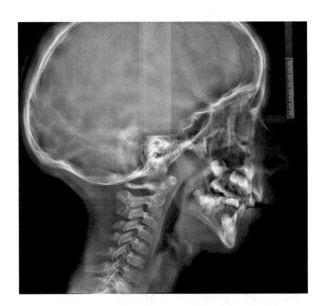

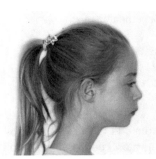
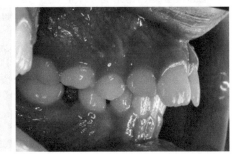

Fig. 4.31 Stickler syndrome

4.6 Orthodontic Ideals

For the tongue to clear adequate oral pharyngeal space, it must sit forward and high into the mouth, resting fully on the palate (Fig. 4.32). Well-formed palates are a mirror image of the dorsum of the tongue as they fully receive the resting tongue (Fig. 4.33). Correctly placed and sized jaws allow the tongue to be housed fully in the closed mouth, the ideal position at rest for optimal pharyngeal airway.

Optimally, in a well-functioning maxillomandibular complex, there will be light wear of teeth with adequate spacing between all teeth in the primary dentition and evenness of alignment in the permanent dentition (Fig. 4.34).

Ideally every organ should be in its place with its own space with even matching of the upper and lower jaw and teeth.

There should be even show off upper and lower teeth with a small gingival display and no dark corridors to the sides in the smile. It is expected there is sufficient room and correct balance in placement for 20 primary teeth and then later for 32 adult teeth (Fig. 4.35).

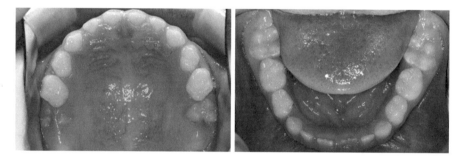

Fig. 4.32 For the tongue to clear adequate oral pharyngeal space, it must sit forward and high into the mouth, resting fully on the palate

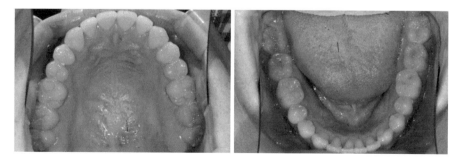

Fig. 4.33 Well-formed palates are a mirror image of the dorsum of the tongue as they fully receive the resting tongue

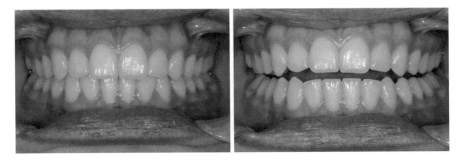

Fig. 4.34 Evenness of alignment in the permanent dentition

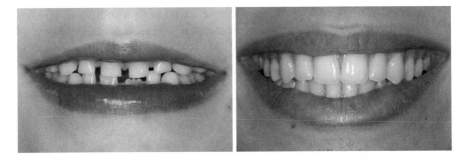

Fig. 4.35 Sufficient room and correct balance in placement for 20 primary teeth and then later for 32 adult teeth

4.7   Treatment Objectives in Obstructive Sleep Apnoea

Breik et al. [36] revealed complete corrections for obstructive sleep apnoea in children with deficient mandibles are possible through distraction osteogenesis. In a similar vein, Hsieh and Lia [37] and Zaghi et al. [38] concluded maxillomandibular advancement to be definitively corrective in adults suffering from obstructive sleep apnoea.

Hsieh et al. [39] observed the anterior movements of the maxilla, soft palate and hyoid in dual jaw surgical advancement cases. The parallel findings of Schendel et al. [40] and Butterfield et al. [41] concluded the resultant creation of increase in pharyngeal airspace was why the mandibular maxillary advancement closing rotation surgery corrects obstructive sleep apnoea.

Iwasaki et al. [42] likely pieced together the explanation of the causal correction from these surgical therapies: linking tongue posture improvement and pharyngeal airway enlargement.

Given this understanding of how facial and dental structures impact airway patency, treatment objects should be aimed to prioritizing development of forward facial growth. Concurrent guarding against retractive interventions must also be allowed for as recommended by Knudesn et al. [43].

For the growing child, in order to safeguard against obstructive sleep apnoea, "counterclockwise closing rotation" upward and forward maxillomandibular development is paramount.

Although the orthodontic profession persist with its view that malocclusion is a genetically driven developmental deviation, it is important to consider that this does not necessarily follow the findings of anthropological and genetic studies. Corruccini [44, 45], Evensen and Ogarrd [46], Jerome et al. [47] and Pinhasi et al. [48] all suggest the role of environmental factors as being significant. Certainly Mossey [49] suggests there is reason to question a purely genetic-based aetiology, and both Uyeda et al. [50] and Cole et al. [51] place the timeline of malocclusion outside the parameters of evolutionary change.

Although it is easy to dismiss the impact of the orthodontic therapy at the basal level, Lundstrom and Woodside [52] demonstrated this has never been true, and significant shifts in growth trends are possible over large numbers of the population undergoing routine treatment. Bork and Skieller [53] also revealed this applies even to the mandible and over an extensive time frame from birth right through to adulthood.

Currently Carvalho et al. [54] supports the use of oral appliance or functional orthopaedic appliance when craniofacial anomalies are present. Villa et al. [55] and Camacho et al. [56] recommend maxillary expansion as effective in improving OSA marker Apnoea-Hypopnoea Index in both the short and long term. Both Camacho et al. [57] and Chuang et al. [58] advocate myofunctional therapy on children with OSA.

Therefore, the common practices to wait until puberty before orthodontic treatment is undertaken can work against the correction of vertical facial growth trends. It is important not to forget the practice of orthodontics accepts dentoalveolar changes are always possible. Remembering the ratio of dentoalveolar to basal bone proportion is not fixed but rather is highest in the early years will give correct justification for interceptive therapies in the first decade of life (Figs. 4.36 and 4.37).

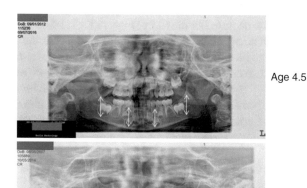

Fig. 4.36 The ratio of dentoalveolar to basal bone proportion is not fixed but rather is highest in the early years will give correct justification for interceptive therapies in the first decade of life

Age 4.5

Age 7

Fig. 4.37 The ratio of dentoalveolar to basal bone proportion is not fixed but rather is highest in the early years will give correct justification for interceptive therapies in the first decade of life

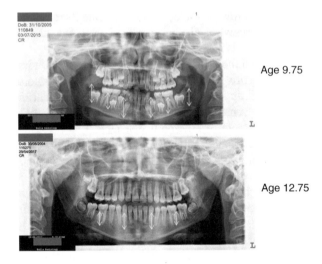

Age 9.75

Age 12.75

4.8   Other Tools of Observation

X-ray comparative of pre- and post-operatively skeletal and dental forms has always been a defining measurement of orthodontic success. Broadening the field of vision to include the soft tissues of the pharyngeal space can be of great service for the management of SDBS. As Neelapu et al. [59] and Momany et al. [60] imply, a greater emphasis on pharyngeal space measurements will redirect focus when diagnosing and revaluating for finishing (Figs. 4.38, 4.39, and 4.40). For modern-day orthodontics to truly thrive in healthcare, vital function must also be considered for when marking for overall success.

Chen et al. [61] suggests an airway centric approach with the use of cone beam computer tomography will allow an even greater view for the interpretation of measurements captured in the films (Figs. 4.41 and 4.42).

Interdisciplinary cross referral is paramount in the total care of the obstructive sleep apnoeic child. Although it is not within the licensure of the dental professional to diagnose any SDBSs, the paediatric dentist or orthodontist may be amongst the first to recognise signs and symptoms that give suspicion for SDBS and OSA. Chervin et al. [62] developed the paediatric sleep questionnaire and Villa et al. [63] the Sleep Clinical Record, both validated to be simple but effective instrument of prediction for general practice medical screening. Ideally the dental profession can also consider incorporating this history-taking form into their routine examination practice and in so doing extend its scope a little further beyond the teeth borders.

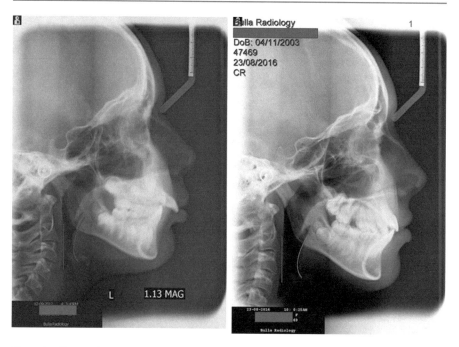

Fig. 4.38 Pre- and post-operative cephalometric X-rays with pharyngeal airway markings. This case is treated using orthotropic (correct growth guidance) therapy

Fig. 4.39 Pre- and post-operative cephalometric X-rays with pharyngeal airway markings. This case is treated using orthotropic (correct growth guidance) therapy

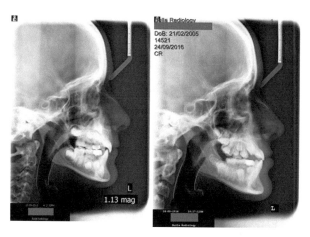

Fig. 4.40 Pre- and post-operative cephalometric X-rays with pharyngeal airway markings. This case is treated using orthotropic (correct growth guidance) therapy

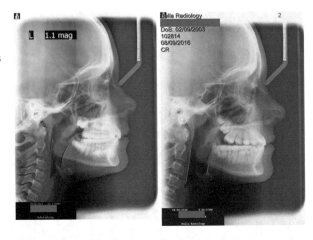

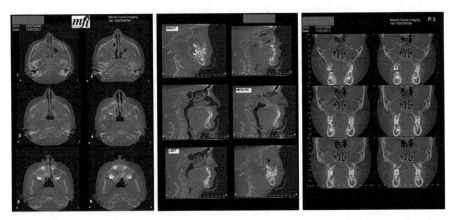

Fig. 4.41 CBCT (cone beam CT) airway evaluation

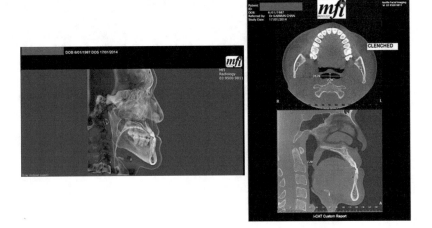

Fig. 4.42 CBCT (cone beam CT) airway evaluation

4.9   Optimized Treatment Outcomes

Ultimately of course redirecting vertical facial growth to a more horizontal trend, irrespective of race, gender or genetics, can be easily seen, as its own measure of aesthetic success (Figs. 4.43, 4.44, 4.45, 4.46, 4.47, 4.48, 4.49, 4.50, 4.51, and 4.52).

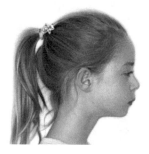
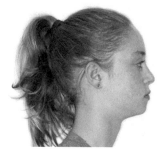

Fig. 4.43 Before and after profile images showing redirecting vertical growth to a more horizontal trend using orthotropic (correct growth) therapy

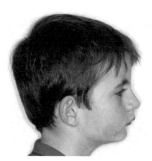
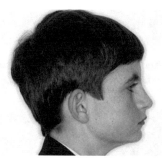

Fig. 4.44 Before and after profile images showing redirecting vertical growth to a more horizontal trend using orthotropic (correct growth) therapy

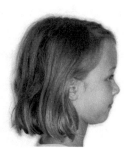
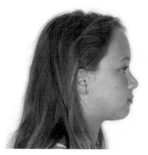

Fig. 4.45 Before and after profile images showing redirecting vertical growth to a more horizontal trend using orthotropic (correct growth) therapy

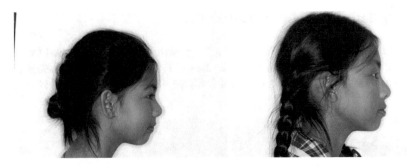

Fig. 4.46 Before and after profile images showing redirecting vertical growth to a more horizontal trend using orthotropic (correct growth) therapy

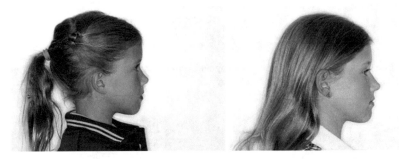

Fig. 4.47 Before and after profile images showing redirecting vertical growth to a more horizontal trend using orthotropic (correct growth) therapy

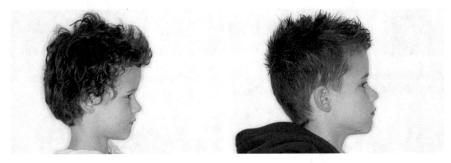

Fig. 4.48 Before and after profile images showing redirecting vertical growth to a more horizontal trend using orthotropic (correct growth) therapy

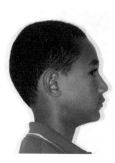
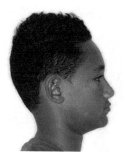

Fig. 4.49 Before and after profile images showing redirecting vertical growth to a more horizontal trend using orthotropic (correct growth) therapy

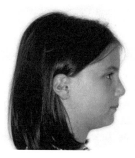
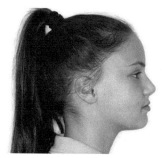

Fig. 4.50 Before and after profile images showing redirecting vertical growth to a more horizontal trend using orthotropic (correct growth) therapy

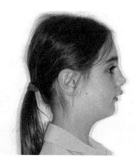
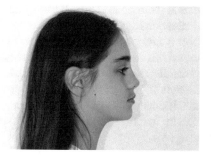

Fig. 4.51 Before and after profile images showing redirecting vertical growth to a more horizontal trend using orthotropic (correct growth) therapy

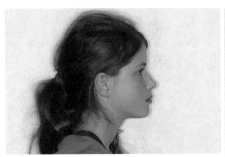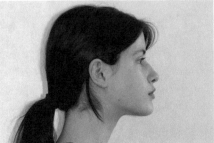

Fig. 4.52 Before and after profile images showing redirecting vertical growth to a more horizontal trend using orthotropic (correct growth) therapy

4.10   Conclusion

Obstructive sleep breathing disorders by definition relate to functional changes in airway patency. The contemporary view draws together deviations with craniofacial growth and development with functional and postural disturbances of the maxillomandibular structures. Readily observable traits in head neck and jaw posture, facial form characteristics of nose shape, eye surrounds, cheek fullness, lip competency/tone, tongue size and tethering as well as breathing and swallow patterns are revealing for deeper disruptions of the upper airway function.

As routine orthodontic evaluations are regularly carried out on children growing with jaw imbalances, opportunities abound to deepen the assessment criteria and search for clues for the airway compromised. The three-dimensional skeletal and dental pictures developed using Angle's and facial height classifications and X-ray evaluations can be broadened further to account for obstructions in the airway. Even observation of commonly seen dental presentations such as narrow palates, crossbites and dental erosion or excessive decay when viewed in the context of sleep breathing disorders is very revealing.

Syndrome malformations present distortions in the extreme of the maxillomandibular complex. These cases readily give acknowledgement; normal breath function requires craniofacial structures to lie within defined boundary ranges.

Awareness of disorders that increasingly plague our children gains true value when management aims to be curative. Surgical corrections to advance the facial complex have been shown to be corrective for obstructive sleep apnoea. It is imperative therefore that these objectives and goals in craniofacial rebalancing become definitive standard of care for all the health professions.

Coupling this understanding with our deeper knowledge in genetics and the relationships between hard and soft body tissue, orthodontic care planning will be expected to expand its impact beyond the aesthetic improvements of the smile. Only by dealing with developmental issues earlier in the timeline will we be able to intervene to prevent craniofacial growth anomalies, reduce the severity of sleep breathing disorders and improve overall vital function for all our children.

References

1. Kaditis AG, et al. Obstructive sleep disordered breathing in 2-18 year old children: diagnosis and management. European Respiratory Society Statement. Eur Respir J. 2016;47:69.
2. Huang YS, Guilleminault C. Pediatric obstructive sleep apnea and the critical role of oral-facial growth: evidences. Front Neurol. 2013;22(3):184.
3. Dibbets JMH. Morphological associations between the Angle classes. Eur J Orthod. 1996;18:111–8.
4. Björk A. The use of metallic implants in the study of facial growth in children: method and application. Am J Phys Anthropol. 1968;29:243–54.
5. Ruf S, Baltromejus S, Pancherz H. Effective condylar growth and chin position changes in activator treatment. Angle Orthod. 2001;71:4–11.
6. McNamara JA. Components of class II malocclusion in children 8–10 years of age. Angle Orthod. 1981;51(3):177–202.
7. Platou C, Zachrisson BU. Incisor position in Scandinavian children with ideal occlusion. Am J Orthod. 1983;83:341–52.
8. Linder-Aronson S. Respiratory function in relation to facial morphology and the dentition. Br J Orthod. 1979;6(2):59–71.
9. Hultcrantz E, Lofstrand T. The development of sleep disorder breathing from 4 to 12 years and dental arch morphology. Int J Pediatr Otorhinolaryngol. 2009;73(9):1234–41.
10. Kim JH, Guilleminault C. The nasomaxillary complex, the mandible and sleep-disordered breathing. Sleep Breath. 2011;15(2):185–93.
11. Migueis DP, et al. Systematic review: the influence of nasal obstruction on sleep apnea. Braz J Otorhinolaryngol. 2016;82:223.
12. Venkamp RP, et al. Tonsillectomy or adenotonsillectomy versus non-surgical management for obstructive sleep disordered breathing in children. Cochrane Database Syst Rev. 2015;(10):CD011165.
13. De Felicio CM, et al. Orofacial motor functions in pediatric obstructive sleep apnea and implications for myofunctional therapy. Int J Pediatr Otorhinolaryngol. 2016;90:5.
14. Glatz-Noll E, Berg R. Oral disfunction in children with Down's Syndrome: an evaluation of treatment effects by means of video-registration. Eur J Orthod. 1991;13:446–51.
15. Trotman C, McNamara J, Dibbets J, van der Weele LT. Association of lip posture and the dimensions of the tonsils and sagittal airway with facial morphology. Angle Orthod. 1997;67:425–32.
16. Luzi V. The CV value (Combined Variation) in the analysis of sagittal malocclusions. Am J Orthod. 1982;81:478–80.
17. Trenouth MJ, Timms DJ. Relationship of the functional oropharynx to craniofacial morphology A random sample of 82 British schoolchildren. Angle Orthod. 1999;69:419–23.
18. Bernabe E, del Castillo CE, Flores-Mirb C. Intra-arch occlusal indicators of crowding in the permanent dentition. Am J Orthod Dentofacial Orthop. 2005;128:220–5.
19. Marcotte MR. Head posture & dento-facial proportion. Angle Orthod. 1981;51:208–15.
20. Vig PS. Experimental manipulation of head posture. Am J Orthod. 1989;77:258–68.
21. Mew JRC. The cause and cure of malocclusion. Heathfield: Brailsham Castle; 2013.
22. Matsuo K, Palmer J. Anatomy and physiology of feeding and swallowing – normal and abnormal. Phys Med Rehabil Clin N Am. 2008;19:691.
23. Van De Engel-Hoek L, et al. Feeding and swallowing disorders in pediatric neuromuscular diseases: an overview. J Neuromusc Dis. 2015;2:357.
24. Machado AJ, et al. Radiographic position of the hyoid bone in children with atypical deglutition. Eur J Orthod. 2012;34:83.
25. Almiro JM, et al. Cephalometric evaluation of the airway space and head posture in children with normal and atypical deglutition: correlations study. Int J Orofacial Myology. 2013;39:69.
26. Brace CK. Egg on the face, f in the mouth, and the overbite. Am Anthropol. 1986;88:695.
27. Mathew JL, Narang I. Sleeping too close together: obesity and obstructive sleep apnea in childhood and adolescence. Paediatr Respir Rev. 2014;15:211.

28. Narang I, Mathew JL. Childhood obesity and obstructive sleep apnea. J Nutr Metab. 2012;2012:134202.
29. Ruanpeng D, et al. Sugar and artificially sweetened beverages linked to obesity: a systematic review and meta analysis. QJM. 2017;110(8):513–20.
30. Flores-Mir C, et al. Craniofacial morphological characteristics in children with obstructive sleep apnea syndrome: a systematic review and meta analysis. JADA. 2013;144(3):269–77.
31. Guilleminault C, Huseni S, Lo L. A frequent phenotype for paediatric sleep apnoea: short lingual frenulum. ERJ Open Res. 2016;2:00043.
32. Noronha AC, et al. Gastroesophageal reflux and obstructive sleep apnea in childhood. Int J Pediatr Otorhinolaryngol. 2009;73:383.
33. Ranjitkar S, Kaidonis J, Smales R. Gastroesophageal reflux disease and tooth erosion. Int J Dent. 2012;2012:479850.
34. Major MP, Flores-Mir C, Major PW. Assessment of lateral cephalometric diagnosis of adenoid hypertrophy and posterior upper airway obstruction: a systematic review. Am J Orthod Dentofacial Orthop. 2006;130(6):700–8.
35. Vieira BB, et al. Cephalometric evaluation of facial pattern and hyoid bone position in children with obstructive sleep apnea syndrome. Int J Pediatr Otorhinolaryngol. 2011;75:383.
36. Breik O, Tivey D, Umapathysivam K, Anderson P. Mandibular distraction osteogenesis for the management of upper airway obstruction in children with micrognathia: a systematic review. Int J Oral Maxillofac Surg. 2016;45:769.
37. Hsieh YJ, Lia YF. Effects of maxillomandibular advancement on the upper airway and surrounding structures in patients with obstructive sleep apnoea: a systematic review. Br J Oral Maxillofac Surg. 2013;51:834.
38. Zaghi S, et al. Maxillomandibular advancement for treatment of obstructive sleep apnea: a meta analysis. JAMA Otolaryngol Head Neck Surg. 2016;142:58.
39. Hsieh YJ, et al. Changes in the calibre of the upper airway and the surrounding structures after maxillomandibular advancement for obstructive sleep apnoea. Br J Oral Maxillofac Surg. 2014;52:445.
40. Schendel SA, Broujerdi JA, Jacobson RL. Three dimensional upper airway changes with maxillomandibular advancement for obstructive sleep apnea treatment. Am J Orthod Dentofacial Orthop. 2014;146:385.
41. Butterfield KJ, et al. Linear and volumetric airway changes after maxillomandibular advancement for obstructive sleep apnea. J Oral Maxillofac Surg. 2015;73:1133.
42. Iwasaki T, et al. Tongue posture improvement and pharyngeal airway enlargement as secondary effects of rapid maxillary expansion: a cone-beam computed tomography study. Am J Orthod Dentofacial Orthop. 2013;143(2):235–45.
43. Knudesn TB, et al. Improved apnea hypopnea index and lowest oxygen saturation after maxillomandibular advancement with or without counterclockwise rotation in patients with obstructive sleep apnea: a meta analysis. J Oral Maxillofac Surg. 2015;73:719.
44. Corruccini RS. An epidemiologic transition in dental occlusion in world populations. Am J Orthod. 1984;86:419.
45. Corruccini RS, et al. Genetic and environmental determinants of dental occlusal variation in twins of different nationalities. Hum Biol. 1990;62:353.
46. Evensen JP, Ogarrd B. Are malocclusions more prevalent and severe now? A comparative study of medieval skulls from Norway. Am J Orthod Dentofacial Orthop. 2007;131(6):710–6.
47. Jerome R, et al. The origins of dental crowding and malocclusions: an anthropological perspective. Compend Contin Educ Dent. 2009;30:292.
48. Pinhasi R, et al. Incongruity between affinity patterns based on mandibular and lower dental dimensions following the transition to agriculture in the Near East, Anatolia and Europe. PLoS One. 2015;10:e0117301.
49. Mossey PA. The heritability of malocclusion: Part 1 Genetics, principles and terminology. Br J Orthod. 1999;26:103–13.
50. Uyeda JC, et al. The million year wait for macro evolutionary bursts. Proc Natl Acad Sci U S A. 2011;108:15908.

51. Cole JB, et al. Human facial shape and size heritability and genetic correlations. Genetics. 2017;205:967.
52. Lundstrom A, Woodside DG. Individual variation in growth directions expressed at the chin and the midface. Eur J Orthod. 1980;2:65.
53. Bork A, Skieller V. Normal and abnormal growth of the mandible. A synthesis of longitudinal cephalometric implant studies over a period of 25 years. Eur J Orthod. 1983;5:1.
54. Carvalho FR, et al. Oral appliances and functional orthopaedic appliances for obstructive sleep apnoea in children. Cochrane Database Syst Rev. 2016;10:CD005520.
55. Villa MP, et al. Efficacy of rapid maxillary expansion in children with obstructive sleep apnea syndrome: 36 months of follow up. Sleep Breath. 2011;15:179–84.
56. Camacho M, et al. Rapid maxillary expansion for pediatric obstructive sleep apnea: a systematic review and meta analysis. Laryngoscope. 2017;127(7):1712–9.
57. Camacho M, et al. Myofunctional therapy to treat obstructive sleep apnea: a systematic review and meta analysis. Sleep. 2015;38(5):669–75.
58. Chuang LC, et al. Passive myofunctional therapy applied on children with obstructive sleep apnea: a 6 month follow up. J Formos Med Assoc. 2017;116:536.
59. Neelapu BC, et al. Craniofacial and upper airway morphology in adult obstructive sleep apnea patients: a systematic review and met analysis of cephalometric studies. Sleep Med Rev. 2017;31:79.
60. Momany SM, et al. Cone beam computed tomography analysis of upper airway measurements in patients with obstructive sleep apnea. Am J Med Sci. 2016;352:376.
61. Chen H, et al. Three dimensional imaging of the upper airway anatomy in obstructive sleep apnea: a systematic review. Sleep Med. 2016;21:19.
62. Chervin RD, et al. Pediatric sleep questionnaire: prediction of sleep apnea and outcomes. Arch Otolaryngol Head Neck Surg. 2007;133:216–22.
63. Villa MP, et al. Sleep clinical record: an aid to rapid and accurate diagnosis of paediatric sleep disorder breathing. Eur Respir J. 2013;41:1355–61.

Physical Assessment in Pediatric Sleep Hygiene and Airway Health

5

Kevin L. Boyd

5.1 Introduction

In addition to *plaque-mediated* dental diseases of childhood, mainly early childhood caries (ECC) and gingivitis, recent evidence suggests that pediatric malocclusion is additionally being recognized as a serious public health dilemma per its frequent comorbid association with sleep and breathing disturbances. Specifically, retrognathic, narrow, excessively vertical, and deficient sagittal skeletal phenotypes in children are often associated with increased risk susceptibility for impaired nasal breathing [1–3].

5.2 Pediatric Sleep Hygiene and Airway Health (p-SAH)

In order to perform a clinically validated appraisal of *pediatric sleep and airway hygiene* (p-SAH) status in a clinical setting, one must collect accurate descriptive data about *physical* traits (e.g., malocclusion phenotypes) known to be commonly associated with p-SAH and *behavioral* traits known to be commonly associated with p-SAH [4], such as sleep-disordered breathing/obstructive sleep apnea (SDB/OSA), parasomnias (e.g., night terrors, bruxism, restless legs, frequent arousals), bedwetting, and diaphoresis. With one exception being morning leg soreness, most p-SAH physical assessment phenotypes are located within the head and neck region, and thus the term *craniofacial*, an adjective referring to the parts of the head containing the brain and the face, is often used as a general address for where one might locate structural deficiencies that could possibly be associated with negative p-SAH. And while many anatomical structures essential to the proper functioning

K. L. Boyd (✉)
Lurie Children's Hospital, Chicago, IL, USA

Private practice, Dentistry for Children, Chicago, IL, USA

© Springer Nature Switzerland AG 2019
E. Liem (ed.), *Sleep Disorders in Pediatric Dentistry*,
https://doi.org/10.1007/978-3-030-13269-9_5

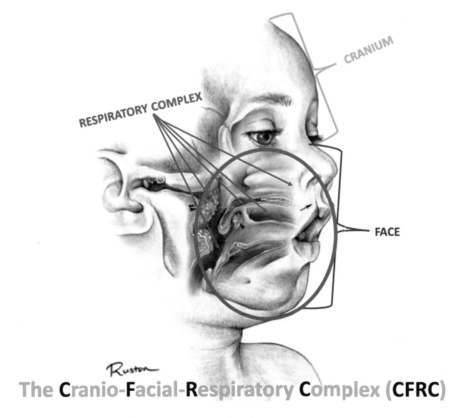

Fig. 5.1 The craniofacial-respiratory complex (CFRC)

of a child's respiratory apparatus are indeed located within and near to the craniofacial area (e.g., mandible, maxilla, anterior nares, nasal valves, nasal septum, tongue, hard palate, lips), other vital respiratory anatomical components are not located there (e.g., soft palate; posterior naso-, oro-, and laryngo-pharynx; posterior nares (choanae); hyoid bone; cervical spine; pharyngeal dilator muscles). So, in the interest of being more inclusive and scientifically accurate, it seems reasonable to suggest that the term *craniofacial-respiratory complex* (CFRC) (Fig. 5.1) rather than *craniofacial* alone would be a more inclusive and useful term for describing precisely where structural deficiencies associated with negative p-SAH might be located.

5.3 Normative Standards

Varieties of malocclusion phenotypes are nearly ubiquitous in industrialized cultures, but seldom seen in cultures that had not yet been exposed to cultural industrialization [5]; similarly, human malocclusion does not appreciably appear in

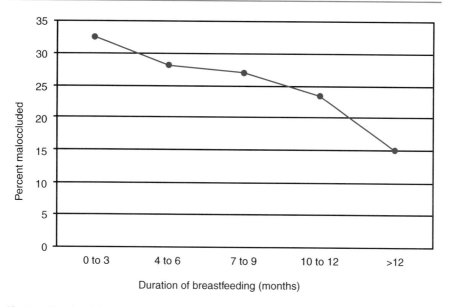

Duration of breastfeeding (months)

Fig. 5.2   Reprinted from Labbok MH, Hendershot GE. Does breast-feeding protect against malocclusion? An analysis of the 1981 Child Health Supplement to the National Health Interview Survey. *Am J Prev Med.* 1987;3(4):227-232

the human fossil and skeletal records until the middle to late eighteenth- century [6]; nursing and weaning practices associated with cultural industrialization seem to be associated with higher prevalence of pediatric malocclusion in so-called *Western-exposed* societies [7] (Fig. 5.2). Established normative standards currently in use today for diagnosing morphological discrepancies of the CFRC (i.e., malocclusion) are largely based upon early to mid-twentieth-century subjective measurements that had been derived from very small data sets [8]. Given what is now well understood about the relative scarcity of human malocclusion phenotypes prior to cultural industrialization [9], to utilize a malocclusion classification system and cephalometric normative standards that had been created from postindustrial samples (i.e., late 19th to mid-twentieth-century Caucasians mostly of European origin) cannot now be considered a scientifically defensible practice. For example, in 1899, E.H. Angle published the paper *Classification of Malocclusion* [10] describing a system of three basic malocclusion phenotypes that is still being utilized today as the *gold standard* for orthodontic diagnosis and treatment. Additionally, in 1953, Cecil Steiner, a former student of E.H. Angle, published *Cephalometrics for You and Me* [11], where he described his *ideal* numeric values as not actually been derived from any sample, but, as he described, "to express our concept of a normal average American child of average age" and also as being useful to his clinical perceptions of therapeutic goals. And finally, a third contribution to the body of orthodontic literature, commonly purported as being a virtual *trilogy* of established craniofacial normative reference standards, was the publication in 1972 by L. Andrews of *The Six Keys to Normal Occlusion* [12], where he described his concept of the *optimal occlusion*

Fig. 5.3 Normally
occluded teeth demonstrate
gingival portion of crown
more distal than occlusal
portion of crown. (After
specimen in possession of
Dr. F. A. Peeso, from
Turner American Textbook
of Prosthetic Dentistry,
Philadelphia, 1913, Lea &
Febiger)

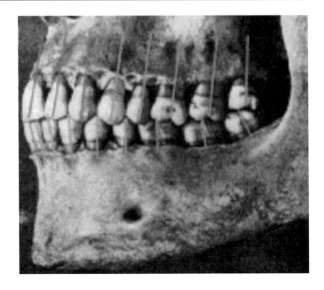

in the permanent dentition as defined by the way certain reference teeth lined up adjacent to and opposed to one another; his data set consisted of 120 study casts from individuals with so-called natural (non-orthodontically treated) *ideal* occlusions. It is interesting to note that Andrews includes an image of a pre-industrial skull (Fig. 5.3) as a prime example of *ideal* crown angulation, the third of his *six keys*.

5.4   Craniofacial-Respiratory Morphology and Pediatric Systemic Health

As mentioned previously, there is ever-accumulating evidence regarding the positive association between maldevelopments of the CFRC in early childhood and risk for susceptibility to negative p-SAH [13]; and while not ethically possible to study prospectively, it seems reasonable to suggest that specific SDB/OSA-associated comorbidities, such as neurological (e.g., ADD/ADHD, cognitive dysfunction.) and peripheral (e.g., appetite hormone dysregulation, type 2 diabetes, impaired somatic growth) systemic illness symptoms, might also be improved in conjunction with appropriate orthodontic/dentofacial orthopedic interventions. It might therefore soon become a medically indefensible position to describe as harmless (i.e., unnecessary to treat) certain malocclusion phenotypes that often first become evident in early childhood (i.e., in the primary/early mixed dentition), such as lack of deciduous interdental spacing or moderate/severe dental crowding, excess vertical, anterior-posterior, sagittal and/or transverse discrepancies, and highly vaulted palates. In addition to the aforementioned inadequacies of the currently used normative standards for what might constitute a healthy/unhealthy CFRC phenotype in early childhood, an additional obstacle to provision of appropriately timed and applied, and often *medically indicated,* early orthodontic intervention is centered around an orthodontic clinician's ability, or inability as might be the case, to manage age-appropriate child anxiety and parental concerns, expectations, and anxiety that are often associated with discussing and receiving *nontraditional* orthodontic treatment (i.e., in the deciduous/early mixed dentition). Specifically, the established curriculum for accredited US postgraduate training programs in orthodontics as is outlined and certified by the American Dental Association's Committee on Dental Accreditation (CODA) [14] fails to require of their resident trainees the appropriate didactic and/or clinical experience in the areas of child emotional development and anxiety management and behavioral guidance in novel healthcare environments. Furthermore, the American Board of Orthodontics does not require candidates to demonstrate any degree of competence in the area of the aforementioned behavior guidance skills in order to become board certified.

5.5 Future Directions

5.5.1 Technology

Over the past two decades, there have been many scientific efforts aimed at understanding how/why optimal p-SAH is vital to overall health and wellness. Recent advances in the sophistication of imaging equipment, such as CBCT, intraoral scanners, and 3-D extra-oral cameras, have improved accuracy and simplified record-taking procedures that are essential for correctly diagnosing and appropriately treating young pediatric patients with malocclusion phenotypes associated with increased SDB/OSA risk. Indisputably the *gold standard* for objectively assessing sleep quantity and quality, is overnight polysomnogram (PSG) sleep studies; however, as PSG testing can be both expensive and physically burdensome to children and their families, aiming to predict OSAS by incorporating data from clinical history and physical examination, various scientifically validated p-SAH screening assessment tools, like the Pediatric Sleep Questionnaire (PSQ) [4] and the Sleep Clinical Record (SCR) [13], have been shown to correlate closely with PSG metrics and thus might serve as reliable substitutes on occasions where overnight PSG testing within a qualified pediatric sleep lab might not be an option. Screening devices like the PSQ and SCR can now be further strengthened with the additional ability to now gather pertinent objective physiological data, such as p-CO_2, HRV, cardiopulmonary coupling, pulse oximetry, and actigraphy, either in-office or at-home when an institutional PSG might not be feasible.

5.6 Cross-Disciplinary Collaboration

According to Stephen Sheldon [16], textbooks in pediatric Sleep Medicine traditionally contain multiple pages describing diseases that children seldom get, but usually contain only a few paragraphs, or at most a few pages, about sleep, which is something that affects the health and wellness of *all* children. Only over recent years has pediatric Sleep Medicine started to become recognized as a scientific discipline that should be understood by *all* allied health professionals who provide care for children. With this knowledge about the importance of how/why children can benefit from attaining optimal SAH as early in their lives as might be deemed feasible, allied health professionals will be able to more easily collaborate with one another in their individual and collective efforts to improve the growth and development of their mutual young patients; the list of qualified healthcare professionals who might potentially collaborate with dental professionals might include, but are certainly not limited to, pediatric Sleep Medicine physicians, pediatricians, pediatric otolaryngologists, myofunctional therapists, chiropractors, speech and language pathologists, school nurses, and school-based psychologists.

5.7   Conclusions

It is problematic that many dental professionals who provide orthodontic services for children are seemingly unable to provide parents/caregivers of young/very young children with incipient malocclusion traits with advice beyond "wait and see" or possibly "save up your money for braces" per the obvious predictability, persistence, and usual worsening of malocclusion beyond the primary dentition. According to orthodontist L.G. Singleton [17], from the vantage point of pediatric dental specialists of his era (circa. 1933), "….the orthodontist who examines the teeth of children from 3 to 5 years of age and presents to the parents a picture of *incipient malocclusion*, is not rendering his full duty to society if he has nothing better to offer than recommendations of delay until the malocclusion becomes objectively apparent when procedures of a mechanical nature may be instituted to correct the defect."; and Dr. Singleton went on to conclude, "The pretenders in orthodontia should be accorded a rude awakening as imposters upon the ethics of the profession and the innocent child should be protected from this form of charlatanism which has become crude enough to verge upon criminality."

Most healthcare professionals are/were not prepared by their undergraduate or postgraduate training programs to be concerned about, or even be cognizant of, the numerous scientifically validated behavioral and physical traits that are known to be indicative of existing comorbid disease or predictive of pediatric SDB/OSA risk susceptibility. The primary consequences of this apparent void in pediatric didactic and clinical healthcare education are at least twofold: First, many of the children now being/having been diagnosed with ADD/ADHD primarily based upon their overlapping behavioral symptoms with SDB/OSA risk are often prescribed powerful stimulants like Ritalin and Adderall, which can lead to abuse and possible additional dependence on other drugs [18]. A second consequence of Sleep Medicine educational under-preparedness is centered around the establishment of *standards of care* within various allied healthcare specialty disciplines that are involved in diagnosing and treating disorders known to be associated with unhealthy sleep. For example, even though there is ample published evidence within peer-reviewed orthodontic and other scientific journals showing that narrow and highly vaulted hard palates, retrusive and vertically developing mandibles, and anterior open-bites are all considered malocclusion phenotypes that can serve as signals for existing or future comorbid airway disease, which in turn can be predictive of increased risk for ADD/ADHD susceptibility, the American Association of Orthodontists (AAO) continues to recommend that children should receive their first orthodontic evaluation not until sometime before the age of 7. Furthermore, the AAO's most recent brochure [19] states that most orthodontic intervention usually commences not until sometime between the ages of 10 and 13. As mentioned earlier in this chapter, antecedents to narrow, vertical, and retrognathic malocclusion phenotypes are usually first detectable in the primary dentition and usually persist and often become more severe later [20]; it seems inconsistent with a preventive philosophy to ignore a disorder in early childhood [21] that might possibly contribute to negative neurological and/or neurobehavioral health consequences down the road. In light of what is now understood about how certain malocclusion phenotypes can predispose a child to negative health consequences known to be associated restricted craniofacial-respiratory growth, and possibly also somatic and neurological development, the demand for orthodontic services at much younger ages than what is now considered *conventional*, that is, between the ages of 9 and 14 years [16], will likely continue to grow and exceed the existing supply of qualified orthodontic specialists. A solution to this disparity might be arrived upon when/if orthodontists, pediatric dentists, and general dentists who provide orthodontic and pediatric preventive and restorative services for children better collaborate not only with one another to assure that their young patients receive accurate diagnostic and appropriately timed and applied orthodontic/dentofacial orthopedic interventions but also with other qualified health professional stakeholders. Medical and dental literature from the mid-nineteenth through the middle twentieth [22–27] centuries attest to the importance of habitual nose-breathing and how collaboration between orthodontists and otolaryngologists, then called *rhinologists*, can lead to positive outcomes for children who suffer from comorbid malocclusion and naso-respiratory incompetence when in the deciduous or early mixed dentition; one might only speculate about precisely why this approach has apparently only recently been *rediscovered*. As it was obviously an effective collaborative strategy back then, it is reasonable to suggest that it will still be an effective collaborative strategy now.

References

1. Juliano M, Ligia ML. Polysomnographic findings are associated with cephalometric measurements in mouth-breathing children. J Clin Sleep Med. 2009;5(6):554.
2. Kawashima S, et al. Cephalometric comparisons of craniofacial and upper airway structures in young children with obstructive sleep apnea syndrome. Ear Nose Throat J. 2000;79(7):499.
3. Seerone A, et al. Risk factors for small pharyngeal airway dimensions in preorthodontic children: a three-dimensional study. Angle Orthod. 2017;87(1):138.
4. Chervin RD, et al. Pediatric sleep questionnaire (PSQ): validity and reliability of scales for sleep-disordered breathing, snoring, sleepiness, and behavioral problems. Sleep Med. 2000;1:21–32.

5. Corruccini RS. An epidemiologic transition in dental occlusion in world populations. Am J Orthod. 1984;86:419–26.
6. Gilbert SF. Ecological developmental biology: developmental biology meets the real world. Dev Biol. 2001;233:1–12.
7. Boyd KL. (R)evolutionary health care, guest editorial. Infant Child Adolesc Nutr. 2012;4(6):32–3.
8. Casko JS, Shepherd WB. Dental and skeletal variation within the range of normal. Angle Orthod. 1984;54:5–17.
9. Gibbons A. An evolutionary theory of dentistry. Science. 2012;336(6084):973–5.
10. Angle EH. Classification of malocclusion. Dental Cosmos. 1899;41(3):248–64.
11. Steiner CC. Cephalometrics for you and me. Am J Orthod. 1953;39:729–55.
12. Andrews LA. The six keys to normal occlusion. Am J Orthod. 1972;62(3):296–309.
13. Boyd KL, Sheldon SH. Sleep disorder breathing: a dental perspective. In: Principles and practice of pediatric sleep medicine. 2nd ed. Amsterdam: Elsevier Inc; 2012. p. 275–80.
14. Commission on Dental Accreditation. Accreditation standards for advanced specialty education programs in orthodontics and dentofacial orthopedics. Accessed 20 Feb 2017, from http://www.ada.org/~/media/CODA/Files/ortho.pdf?la=en.
15. Pilla Via M, et al. Diagnosis of pediatric obstructive sleep apnea syndrome in settings with limited resources. JAMA Otolaryngol Head Neck Surg. 2015;141(11):990–6.
16. Personal communication with this author.
17. Singleton LG. The human side of orthodontia. Angle Orthod. 1934;4(4):305–11.
18. Keane H. Pleasure and discipline in the uses of Ritalin. Int J Drug Policy. 2007;19:401–9.
19. American Association of Orthodontists. Your child's first orthodontic checkup. AAO promotional brochure. Accessed 20 Feb 2017, from https://mylifemysmile.org/mylifemysmile/brochures/Your_Childs_First_Checkup.pdf.
20. Baccetti T, et al. Early dentofacial features of Class II malocclusion: a longitudinal study from the deciduous through the mixed dentition. Am J Orthod. 1997;111(5):502–9.
21. Rubin RM. The orthodontist's responsibility in preventing facial deformity. In: McNamara J, editor. Naso-respiratory function and craniofacial growth, Craniofacial growth series, vol. 9. Ann Arbor, MI, Center for Human Growth and Development; 1979.
22. Whiting GF. Mouth-breathing and its Attendant Evils. Dental Cosmos. 1883;25(6):295–306.
23. Pullen HA. Mouth-breathing. Dental Cosmos. 1906;48(10):998–1014.
24. Haskin WH. The relief of nasal obstruction by orthodontia-A plea for early recognition and correction of faulty maxillary development. Laryngoscope. 1912;22(11):1237–60.
25. Bogue EA. Enlargement of the nasal sinuses in young children by orthodontia. J Am Med Assoc. 1909;53(6):441–4.
26. Cohen SA. Malocclusion and its far reaching effects. J Am Med Assoc. 1922;79(23):1895–7.
27. Bogue EA. The position of the deciduous teeth, an important diagnostic symptom. Int J Orthodon Oral Surg. 1921;7(5):237–50.

Airway Orthodontics, the New Approach

6

Barry D. Raphael

This purpose of this chapter is to discuss the therapeutic or behavioral interventions that can be a part of a preventive approach to sleep-disordered breathing.

6.1 Introduction

No one would deny that many of the factors that lead up to a coronary blockage can be addressed by either therapeutic or behavioral interventions and that, certainly, prevention is a far better choice. But there has been an absence of such discussion regarding occlusion of the airway. The purpose of this chapter is to stimulate such a discussion and to paint a picture of what a preventive approach to sleep-disordered breathing would look like.

6.2 The Etiology and Predisposition to Breathing Disorders During Sleep

It was once thought that obstructive sleep apnea was a disease of old, fat men. We have since learned that thin, athletic women can also fall victim to this problem as well as children. We have learned that while weight and age add to the susceptibility to obstructive sleep disorders, they are not the root causes. Difficulty breathing at night comes from resistance to airflow, and there are many circumstances that can make breathing difficult. Efforts at pinpointing the source of resistance are important to determining proper remediation.

B. D. Raphael (✉)
Raphael Center for Integrative Orthodontics, Clifton, NJ, USA
e-mail: drbarry@alignmine.com

E. Liem (ed.), *Sleep Disorders in Pediatric Dentistry*,
https://doi.org/10.1007/978-3-030-13269-9_6

Fig. 6.1 The causes of
airway turbulence

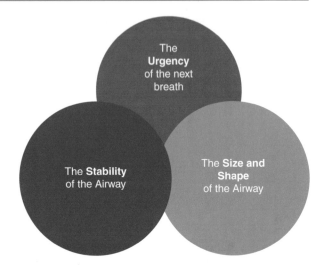

We have learned from flow physics and airway physiology that there are three main determinants of airway resistance:

1. The size and shape of the airway (Anatomy)
2. The stability of the airway (Physiology)
3. The velocity and turbulence of the airflow (Behavior)

Delving into the physics of each is not the point of the chapter. Instead, the way that each of these factors can be addressed well before the first apnea ever occurs with either therapeutic or behavioral interventions will be the goal. By defining opportunities to mitigate predisposing risk factors to airway resistance, we can begin to build a new paradigm in airway and sleep management. As such, the focus will be on prevention so that, just as we might prevent the heart attack, the end-stage disease of obstructive sleep apnea might never occur. From this discussion, a new field of Airway Dentistry and Orthodontics will emerge that can define a possible future for the way orthodontics is practiced (Fig. 6.1).

6.3   Anatomy: The Size and Shape of the Airway

Yes, losing weight and reducing fat deposits in the neck or removing tonsils are widely regarded as important, but we also know that *craniofacial morphology* is a primary risk factor for breathing problems as well [1–4]. Orthodontics has long been concerned with the growth and development of the face with regard to facial profile and the correction of skeletal and dental malocclusion but has only recently considered its relevance to the formation of the naso-oropharyngeal airway [5]. Anatomically, the maxilla (and the soft palate that hangs off the back of it) and the mandible (with the tongue attached to it) create the anterior boundaries of the pharyngeal airway. Studies have shown how retroposition of these bones relative to the face narrow the airway and create the risk for obstruction [2, 6]. This is true in both adults and children. Orthopedic treatments in children are now being explored to help enlarge or at least prevent further restriction of the airway in a more natural and permanent way [7].

Most of the focus in orthopedic research has been on palatal expansion, with the purpose of widening the nasal aperture and palate, with equivocal results [8, 9]. Additionally, studies show that bringing either or both jaws forward with advancement appliances or orthognathic surgery can be effective in opening the airway in the adult [10]. We also know helping either jaw grow forward in the child may also be helpful [11]. More recent work shows that changing maxillary growth in all three planes of space, including advancement, provides even more promising results [7].

Playing off findings in the anthropology literature, the shape of the maxilla has changed dramatically in the modern human. This transformation is associated with a rapid change in the following environmental challenges, all of which have become rampant in today's world: [12]

- Dietary (high sugar and refined carbohydrate content)
- Metabolic (autonomic and digestive stressors)
- Cultural (early feeding and weaning habits)
- Breathing (open mouth and low tongue postures)
- Postural (forward head and slumped shoulders; portable electronics)
- Sleep (artificial light and altered sleep cycles)
- Inflammatory (a changing gut biome)

Given the rapidity of the environmental change, purely genetic variations must be ruled out.

Epigenetic variations of the bone's shape, however, indicate that it is changing in width, yes, but also slumping downward and failing to fill out sagittally as well, a condition being called craniofacial dystrophy [12]. This nearly universal midface deficiency (no matter the Angle classification of the teeth) has formed a bone with a collapsing palate with insufficient room for the teeth, and that often restricts the forward growth of the mandible hampering proper positioning of the tongue all of which limit the eventual size of the airway.

Helping the jaws grow *forward*, not just wider, is the goal. Reversal of midface collapse presents numerous challenges to current orthodontic paradigms that often look to retract teeth and jaws distally (=caudally), but it also empowers us as well. There has been a thread of thought throughout the historical orthodontic literature supporting the idea that a palate is not just congenitally narrow, but *becomes narrow as a result of what we DO*.

Altering these habits can begin to heal the dystrophy.

If the modern lifestyle can create these changes to the modern face so rapidly (in the past 300–400 years), then human ingenuity can reverse them as well. Originally independently formulated by forward thinking clinicians like George Crozat [13], Edward Angle, John Mew, and Chris Farrel, protocols such as Crozat, Advanced Lightwire Functionals, Postural Orthodontics, Biobloc Orthotropics, Cranial Osteopathy, and Myofunctional Orthodontics, all seek to reverse the conditions that lead to midface collapse. All these approaches have a common goal of reestablishing postural support of the growing maxilla by maintaining the resting tongue on the palate as a scaffold for the growing (and non-growing) bone.

The protocols that encourage forward growth of the jaws have all found some measure of success in reducing sleep-disordered breathing [7, 13, 14]. Furthermore, treatments that restrict forward growth or reduce the size of space for the tongue have been shown to reduce airway size and, for purposes of breathing, should be avoided [15].

More research in this area is needed, but common sense says that any technique that enlarges the airway space will be helpful in combating breathing problems.

6.4   Physiology: The Stability of the Airway

Even a fairly substantial airway can be closed off if the walls cannot withstand the turbulence created by the airflow within it. There are several points along the way from the nose to the trachea where soft tissue is apt to give way to the negative pressure (see Fig. 6.2). And there are several conditions that can decrease the stability and increase the collapsibility of these tissues, all of which are reversible to some extent.

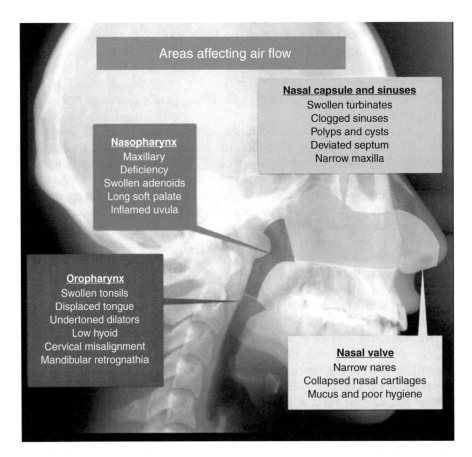

Fig. 6.2 Areas of flow limitation

1. Swelling of lymphoid tissue is perhaps the most commonly recognized problem [16]. Tonsils and adenoids are currently thought of as the predominant risk factor for sleep-disordered breathing in children. The American Academy of Pediatrics has recently stated that surgical removal of lymphoid tissue can be considered a first line of treatment in obstructive sleep apnea [17]. But one question that is rarely asked is, **why** do lymphoid tissues get so swollen as to block the airway in the first place? While they are known to be more reactive in a young growing child, their enlargement, like the collapse of the palate, is not a congenital given. Efforts to reduce the swelling can sometimes dramatically open the airway and may reduce the need for surgery.

   Some of the methods used to reduce lymphoid swelling include:
   (a) A transition from mouth breathing, which allows unfiltered air to irritate the tonsils, to nasal breathing, which filters and conditions the air before it gets to the lymph tissue, can reduce swelling within weeks.
   (b) Improvements in body posture and muscular movement, as with regular exercise, can also help lymph tissue drain adequately.
   (c) A transition from accessory muscle use to proper use of the diaphragm for breathing also helps lymphatic circulation.
   (d) Nasal lavage to keep sinuses open and airway walls clean can help.
   (e) Massage and bodywork can help lymphatic circulation.
   (f) Acupuncture and homeopathic remedies that encourage drainage of lymph tissue throughout the body.
   (g) The use of ozone and ozonated water injected into the swollen tissue has been shown to reduce lymph swelling.
   (h) Short-term use of nasal steroids and decongestions as a good head-start are helpful.

      Certainly, it's better to try to shrink swollen lymph tissues as a preliminary approach. The frequent recurrences seen after surgical removal are probably linked to a failure to incorporate some of the above conservative measures postsurgically, especially continued oral breathing. This makes a conservative approach even more important not only as a first line of defense but also when the tissues are removed.

2. Poor muscle tone is also associated with blockage of the airway. Certainly, the tongue falling back into the oral cavity at night is well recognized as a risk factor for sleep-disordered breathing. But well-toned extrinsic and intrinsic glossal muscles resist backward displacement. The use of myofunctional therapy, with specific exercises for creating better muscular balance of the pharyngeal musculature, has been shown to be helpful in reducing airway collapse at night and deserves more attention in this field [18]. Even learning to play the Australian didgeridoo has been shown to be helpful in reducing pharyngeal collapse at night [19].

3. Chronic inflammation of pharyngeal tissues makes them less able to resist negative pressure due to loss of elasticity. The constant trauma to the tissues of the flapping of snoring only serves to irritate, elongate, and soften pharyngeal tissues and the soft palate. Chronic assault by stomach acid from gastric or laryngeal reflux is another source of inflammation that needs to be addressed.

The cause of reflux itself can be addressed by changes in breathing mode (i.e., nasal breathing) and posture, too, thereby reducing reliance on protein pump inhibitors that have their own side effects. Finally, honing in on foods—some natural, some not—that instigate inflammation or disturb the natural flora in the gut and supplanting them with healthier choices can change the condition of the airway as well as the rest of the body.

6.5   Behavior: Velocity and Turbulence of the Airflow

Though the way air flows through the breathing space has been tested and studied and recognition of air pressure changes within the pharynx and within the thoracic cavity has been given due consideration, little attention has been paid to the behaviors that actually create these negative pressure conditions. In fact, some theorize that it is not the nighttime breathing that creates the biggest problem but the daytime habits of breathing that set up the circumstances for airway collapse at night [20]. These conditions include habitual over-breathing in response to the many chronic stressors that we encounter each day.

Chronic stress has a person adopting certain compensatory behaviors simply because *the urgency to take the next breath* is the most important thing we do moment to moment. The autonomic nervous system is frequently activated without adequate chance for recuperation, setting in motion a cascade of events that result in, among many other things, rapid shallow breathing with tidal volumes nearly three times what is necessary for efficient oxygenation—in other words: chronic hyperventilation.

It is said that over-breathing is just as dangerous to health as overeating. Chronic hyperventilation, especially with the large portal of an open mouth, shifts the balance between oxygen and carbon dioxide in the lungs and in the blood. Chronic hypocapnia (low native stores of carbon dioxide) is a common condition in mouth breathers and can result in reduced oxygenation of tissues (the Bohr effect) and increased smooth muscle spasm (think: vessels and organs). The symptoms from these two phenomena alone are quite diverse, affecting the vasculature (hypertension, venous pooling); organs (enuresis, digestive issues); tubes (asthma, reflux, xerostomia); and tissue perfusion (intermittent hypoxia to the brain, neurocognitive deficits such as attention, memory and learning, anxiety, and muscle fatigue and spasm). And, oh yes, apnea.

Heavy breathing at night pulls air through the pharynx rapidly, creating increased turbulence and negative pressure. This can compromise an otherwise healthy system (e.g., snoring only when you get intoxicated). Combine that with small airway size and you get the perfect internal storm—a hurricane in a box, if you will.

Some think that central sleep apnea is nothing more than the body's respiratory mechanism taking a pause to restore proper carbon dioxide levels and maintain homeostasis. While this thinking seems to be in direct opposition to the commonly held view that sleep-disordered breathing is a problem of hypoventilation and hypercapnia, a change in daytime breathing mode—again, from oral to light nasal breathing—can reduce nighttime distress almost immediately in some patients [21]. In fact, the relationship between daytime breathing habits and nighttime distress is so strong the syndrome should be called breathing-disordered sleep instead of sleep-disordered breathing. Adopting new changes in daytime breathing behaviors should be the first line of defense in the treatment of breathing-disordered sleep.

Simple breathing training includes:

1. Adopt nasal breathing primarily, even during activity, as much as possible.
2. Reduction of tidal volume by reducing breathing rate and depth.
3. Use of the diaphragm for powering inspiration.

Biofeedback techniques are especially helpful in retraining daytime breathing. Once the body can accommodate to this new breathing mode, there is often no longer such a struggle at night. And at very least, modalities like PAP (positive airway pressure) and MADs (mandibular advancement device) can become more tolerable.

6.6   Airway-Related Craniofacial Dysfunctions: A Change in Paradigm

Besides sleep apnea, there are a host of refractory conditions that dentistry has been struggling with that are now being looked upon as airway-related craniofacial dysfunctions (ACDs).

They include:

1. Chronic naso-pharyngeal obstruction (physical or functional) [22]
2. Tethered oral tissues (lip-tie and tongue-tie) [23]
3. Open mouth rest posture (with the tongue off the palate) [24]
4. Myofunctional disorders (swallowing, chewing, etc.) [25]
5. Chronic hyperventilation and hypocapnia [26]
6. Breathing-disordered sleep (OSA, UARS, snoring) [27]
7. Bruxism, parafunctions, and dental deterioration [21]
8. TMD and facial pain components [28]
9. Cranial and postural issues [29]
10. Craniofacial dystrophy with malocclusion [30]

Each topic deserves its own discussion, but putting them under the umbrella of airway dysfunctions seems to have answered a lot of challenging questions for practitioners in all disciplines. In fact, once you see the relationship, it's hard to see how we ever thought otherwise.

6.7   Conclusions and the Future of Orthodontics

The current gold-standard treatment, if gold is the appropriate color, for obstructive sleep apnea is to artificially pry open the airway at night with air, plastic, or scalpel. Perhaps someday we'll have Swarovski-studded tracheostomy plugs for a more perfect (read: fashionable and quick) solution.

Fig. 6.3 Timeline

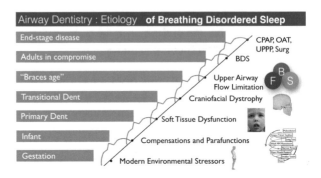

But if you look at the progression of events leading up to obstruction (Fig. 6.3), there are many, many opportunities to intervene, to change the trajectory of the disease and to increase the quality of life. By helping the airway to grow larger (size and shape), keeping the airway physically fit (stability), and optimizing the airway's use (flow), the problem can be, at worst, delayed and, at best, avoided [31].

In recent years, the orthodontic profession has been arguing about the relative benefits of early orthodontic treatment asking, "Is the benefit worth the burden?" [32, 33] One could ask the same question about the effort needed to prevent heart disease. Yet, today, fitness centers and whole foods establishments are becoming mainstream in our society answering that question by popular demand. Perhaps in days soon to come, there will be similar outcry looking for orthodontists and dentists to help adults and children have better sleep and breathing as well. Our job will be to first make the airway easier to breathe through and then to teach children how to breathe easier.

"...craniofacial morphology
is a primary risk factor for
breathing problems..."

"...over-breathing is
just as dangerous to
health as is overeating."

References

1. Aihara K, Oga T, Harada Y, Chihara Y, Handa T, Tanizawa K, Watanabe K, Hitomi T, Tsuboi T, Mishima M, Chin K. Analysis of anatomical and functional determinants of obstructive sleep apnea. Sleep Breath. 2012;16(2):473–81.
2. Dempsey JA, Skatrud JB, Jacques AJ, Ewanowski SJ, Woodson BT, Hanson PR, Goodman B. Anatomic determinants of sleep-disordered breathing across the spectrum of clinical and nonclinical male subjects. Chest. 2002;122(3):840–51.

3. Lowe AA, Santamaria JD, Fleetham JA, Price C. Facial morphology and obstructive sleep apnea. Am J Orthod Dentofacial Orthop. 1986;90(6):484–91.
4. Ikävalko T, Tuomilehto H, Pahkala R, Tompuri T, Laitinen T, Myllykangas R, Vierola A, Lindi V, Närhi M, Lakka TA. Craniofacial morphology but not excess body fat is associated with risk of having sleep-disordered breathing—The PANIC Study (a questionnaire-based inquiry in 6–8-year olds). Eur J Pediatr. 2012;171(12):1747–52.
5. Carlyle TD, Chmura L, Damon P, Diers N, Paquette D, Quintero JC, Redmond WR, Thomas B. Orthodontic strategies for sleep apnea. Orthod Prod. 2014;21(3):92–101. Accessed on April 13, 2016, from http://www.orthodonticproductsonline.com/2014/04/orthodontic-strategies-sleep-apnea/.
6. Katyal V, Pamula Y, Martin AJ, Daynes CN, Kennedy JD, Sampson WJ. Craniofacial and upper airway morphology in pediatric sleep-disordered breathing: Systematic review and meta-analysis. Am J Orthod Dentofacial Orthop. 2013;143(1):20–30.
7. Singh GD, Garcia-Motta AV, Hang WM. Evaluation of the posterior airway space following Biobloc therapy: geometric morphometrics. Cranio. 2007;25(2):84–9.
8. Rose E, Schessl J. Orthodontic procedures in the treatment of OSA in children. J Orofac Orthop. 2006;67(1):58–67.
9. Ruoff CM, Guilleminault C. Orthodontics and sleep-disordered breathing. Sleep Breath. 2012;16(2):271–3.
10. Holty JE, Guilleminault C. Maxillomandibular advancement for the treatment of obstructive sleep apnea: a systematic review and meta-analysis. Sleep Med Rev. 2010;14(5):287–97.
11. Kaygisiz E, Tuncer BB, Yüksel S, Tuncer C, Yildiz C. Effects of maxillary protraction and fixed appliance therapy on the pharyngeal airway. Angle Orthod. 2009;79(4):660–7.
12. Boyd KD. Dentistry: an evolutionary perspective on the etiology of malocclusion, part 1. J Am Orthod Soc. 2011:34–9.
13. Rogers AP. Stimulating arch development by the exercise of the masseter-temporal group of muscles. Am J Orthod Dentofacial Orthop. 1922;8(2):61–4. (originally in The International Journal of Orthodontia, Oral Surgery and Radiography.)
14. Oktay H, Ulukaya E. Maxillary protraction appliance effect on the size of the upper airway passage. Angle Orthod. 2008;78(2):209–14.
15. Villa MP, Bernkopf E, Pagani J, Broia V, Montesano M, Ronchetti R. Randomized controlled study of an oral jaw positioning appliance for the treatment of obstructive sleep apnea in children with malocclusion. Am J Respir Crit Care Med. 2002;165(1):123–7.
16. Wang Q, Jia P, Anderson NK, Wang L, Lin J. Changes of pharyngeal airway size and hyoid bone position following orthodontic treatment of Class I bimaxillary protrusion. Angle Orthod. 2012;82(1):115–21.
17. Li AM, Wong E, Kew J, Hui S, Fok TF. Use of tonsil size in the evaluation of obstructive sleep apnea. Arch Dis Child. 2002;87(2):156–9.
18. Marcus CL, Brooks LJ, Draper KA, Gozal D, Halbower AC, Jones J, Schechter MS, Ward SD, Sheldon SH, Shiffman RN, Lehmann C, Spruyt K. Diagnosis and management of childhood obstructive sleep apnea syndrome. Pediatrics. 2012;130(3):3714–55.
19. Pitta DBS, Pessoa AF, Sampaio ALL, Rodrigues RN, Tavares MG, Tavares P, et al. Oral Myofunctional therapy applied on two cases of severe obstructive sleep apnea syndrome. Int Arch Otorhinolaryngol. 2007;11(3):350–4.
20. Puhan MA, Suarez A, Lo Cascio C, Zahn A, Heitz M, Braendli O. Didgeridoo playing as alternative treatment for obstructive sleep apnoea syndrome: randomized controlled trial. BMJ. 2006;332(7536):266–70.
21. Litchfield PM. Respiratory fitness and acid-base regulation. Psychophysiol Today. 2010;7(1):6–12. Accessed on April 13, 2016, from http://betterphysiology.com/download/softwareupdates/Respiratory%20Fitness%202010%20Litchfield2.pdf.
22. Birch M. Sleep apnoea: a survey of breathing retraining. Aust Nurs J. 2012;20(4):40–1.
23. Chandra RK, Patadia MO, Raviv J. Diagnosis of nasal airway obstruction. Otolaryngol Clin North Am. 2009;42(2):207–25.

24. Kotlow L. infant reflux and aerophagia associated with the maxillary lip-tie and ankyloglossia (tongue-tie). Clin Lactat. 2011;2(4):25–9.
25. Mew M. Craniofacial dystrophy: a possible syndrome? Br Dent J. 2014;216(10):555–8.
26. Guimarães KC, Drager LF, Genta PR, Marcondes BF, Lorenzi-Filho G. Effects of oropharyngeal exercises on patients with moderate obstructive sleep apnea syndrome. Am J Respir Crit Care Med. 2009;179(10):962–6.
27. Ritz T, Meuret AE, Wilhelm FH, Roth WT. Changes in pCO2, symptoms, and lung function of asthma patients during capnometry-assisted breathing training. Appl Psychophysiol Biofeedback. 2009;34(1):1–6.
28. Hosoya H, Kitaura H, Hashimoto T, Ito M, Kinbara M, Deguchi T, Irokawa T, Ohisa N, Ogawa H, Takano-Yamamoto T. Relationship between sleep bruxism and sleep respiratory events in patients with obstructive sleep apnea syndrome. Sleep Breath. 2014;18(4):837–44.
29. Gelb ML. Airway centric TMJ philosophy. J Calif Dent Assoc. 2014;4(8):551–62.
30. James GA, Strokon D. An introduction to cranial movement and orthodontics. Int J Orthod Milwaukee. 2005;16(1):23–6.
31. Huang YS, Guilleminault C. Pediatric obstructive sleep apnea and the critical role of oral-facial growth: evidences. Front Neurol. 2013;22(3):184.
32. Campbell C, Jacobson H. Whole: rethinking the science of nutrition. Dallas, TX: BenBella Books; 2013.
33. McNamara J, editor. Early orthodontic treatment: is the benefit worth the burden? Ann Arbor, MI: University of Michigan Press; 2007.

Orthodontic and Dentofacial Orthopedic Treatment Strategies for Pediatric Sleep Disorders

Edmund A. Lipskis

7.1 Introduction

As early as 1868, Danish otorhinolaryngologist Wilhelm Meyer observed that children with sleep-related breathing issues presented with different facial growth patterns and forms, when compared to children who did not have these disturbances [1]. In 1906, H. A. Pullen published an article discussing the association of mouth breathing with abnormal facial development [2]. At a meeting of the European Orthodontia Society in 1913, Daniel M'Kenzie discusses the problems of mouth breathing and its cure. He attributes the difficulty physicians have, in changing the breathing mode, to structural changes in the maxilla, and discusses a previous article in which he theorized that inferior tongue position found in mouth breathers was at least partly the cause of the palatal deformation he described [3]. In what is today seen by many as classic papers on the topic of changes in facial growth as a result of impaired respiration, Egil Harvold, in 1973 and 1981, published studies which demonstrated modifications in facial growth to accommodate forced mouth breathing in primates [4, 5]. Timo Peltomaki discusses the consequences of OSA and mouth breathing, including increased vertical growth of the face, decreased mandibular growth, and alterations in growth hormone levels affecting the growth of the face along with affecting somatic growth [6]. These studies, along with many others [7–9], describing changes in facial growth in response to airway and breathing issues, have led to highly debated controversies in orthodontics about the importance of respiratory mode in malocclusions and craniofacial form, along with a heated debate about whether early treatment is needed.

As recently as 2014, Anmol Kalha, arguing against early treatment, wrote that reducing incisor trauma in Class II overjet cases was the reason for early orthodontic interventional treatment and that "There appear to be no other advantages for providing treatment early when compared to treatment in adolescence" [10]. For

E. A. Lipskis (✉)
The Centre for Integrative Orthodontics, St. Charles, IL, USA

© Springer Nature Switzerland AG 2019
E. Liem (ed.), *Sleep Disorders in Pediatric Dentistry*,
https://doi.org/10.1007/978-3-030-13269-9_7

those who recognize skeletal problems in children, their relationship to airways and disturbed sleep, and the consequences of not treating early, the dismissal of early treatment seems to disregard important and vital issues that can have lasting or permanent negative consequences for the life of these patients. In a review of the evidence on the role of oral-facial growth and pediatric obstructive sleep apnea, Huang and Guilleminault concluded that pediatric OSA in nonobese children is a disorder of oral-facial growth and that dentofacial orthopedics and orthodontics have a clear positive impact on pediatric OSA [11]. These same conclusions have been reached by many investigators [12–14]. In addition to these findings, many investigators have connected childhood sleep apnea to, among other things, cognitive dysfunction and behavioral disorders [15–17]. Ann Halbower at Johns Hopkins has linked childhood sleep apnea to lower IQ and brain damage, finding altered ratios of neurochemicals indicating damage to brain cells of children with sleep apnea [18]. There is a concern and argument for early treatment of these patients simply by looking at neural development in childhood.

The Harvard Center on the Developing Child has published illustrating the accelerated development of neural pathways, including pathways for cognitive function, in childhood. As can be seen on the graph (Fig. 7.1), the accelerated growth rate for neural pathways associated with higher cognitive function slows down to an adult rate by around age 14. In a 2006 paper discussing the association between childhood OSA and neurocognitive defects and brain injury, Dr. Halbower concludes that sleep apnea in a child treated too late could "permanently alter the trajectory of a developing child's ultimate cognitive potential, resulting in a lifetime of health and economic impacts" [19]. Treatment would need to allow enough time for recovery, so the usual orthodontic treatment times, corresponding to the eruption of the second molars, would likely be too late for full reversal of the cognitive and executive function defects.

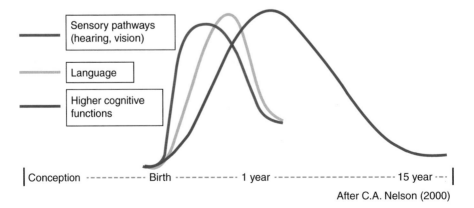

Human brain development

Neural connections for different functions develop sequentially

After C.A. Nelson (2000)

Fig. 7.1 Human brain development

The first line of treatment for pediatric OSA has been adenotonsillectomy [20]. Unfortunately, studies have demonstrated that long-term improvements in airways and in elimination of OSA in children have not resulted from these, as stand-alone procedures, with lasting improvement rates ranging from 32% to 6.7% maintaining acceptable levels of improvement. The percentages are even worse if the initial problem was ranked as moderate or severe apnea, with Ron Mitchell stating "Severe preoperative OSA is associated with persistence of OSA after Adenotonsillect-omy. Postoperative reports of symptoms such as snoring and witnessed apneas correlate well with persistence of OSA after Adenotonsillectomy" [21–23]. It has been found that there are adjunct procedures that can enhance, or even replace, adenotonsillectomy in treating pediatric OSA.

7.2 Orthodontic and Dentofacial Orthopedic Strategies that Affect Craniofacial Structure

7.2.1 Palatal Expansion

There has been a significant amount of research demonstrating improvement in upper airways through palatal expansion, including reduction of AHI scores to normal levels [24–27]. It seems that proper nasal breathing is one of the most key components in the elimination of obstructive sleep apnea. Dr. Christian Guilleminault has stated in a 2014 paper that "Elimination of oral breathing, i.e., restoration of nasal breathing during wake and sleep, may be the only valid endpoint when treating OSA" [28]. It has been the author's observation that enlarged adenoids are not the only finding leading to reduced patency of nasal airways and mouth breathing. With CBCT imaging, it has become quite apparent that nasal airways are generally inadequate in this patient population. This has also been frequently documented in the literature [29, 30]. Reliance and accuracy of CBCT imaging in airway evaluation has also been validated [31]. The treatment strategy of palatal expansion is the most frequently employed dentofacial orthopedic technique employed by orthodontic practitioners in treating pediatric OSA. While most research discusses rapid maxillary expansion (RME), studies have demonstrated that slow maxillary expansion (SME) is equal to or better than RME in expanding the palate in dimension, effect on the nasal airway, and stability [32–34]. These studies also demonstrate that the technique utilized is more important than the appliance selected. There is also mounting evidence that the midpalatal suture remains viable, not ossified, well into adulthood [35] and that there are needed functional reasons for it to not fuse [36]. In order to preserve the integrity of the midpalatal suture, SME is recommended. As Dr. William Proffit has stated in *Contemporary Orthodontics*, "Thus the overall result of rapid vs. slow expansion is similar, but with slower expansion a more physiologic response is obtained" [37]. A case of expansion alone is illustrated below (Figs. 7.2, 7.3, 7.4, 7.5, 7.6, 7.7, and 7.8). Pretreatment HST revealed an AHI of 5.8; post expansion alone the HST showed a drop in AHI to 0. His treatment consisted simply of treatment with an upper Hyrax and a lower "E" spring lateral arch development appliance. Some of his case records are shown:

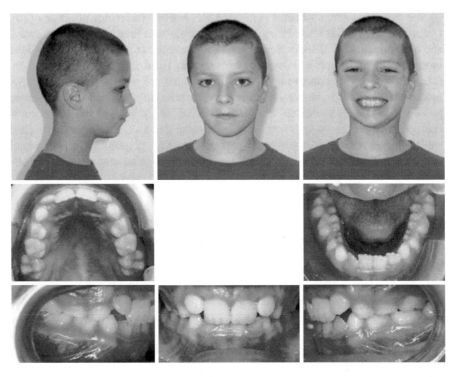

Fig. 7.2 Pretreatment photographs

Fig. 7.3 Upper appliance in place

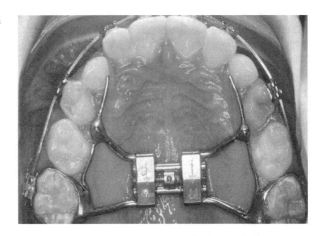

The recommended rate for SME in children is 1/2 mm per week, accomplished by advancing the screw 1/4 mm, twice per week, divided as evenly as possible. In our practice, just for standardization, we have patients activate their appliances on Wednesdays and Sundays. Lower appliances, when activated by a screw-type appliance, should only be activated 1/4 mm per week, still divided into two 1/8 mm

Fig. 7.4 Lower appliance in place

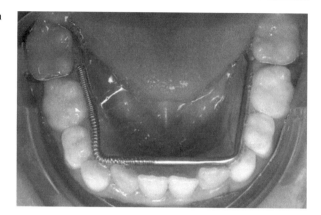

Fig. 7.5 Cross-sectional view of mandible

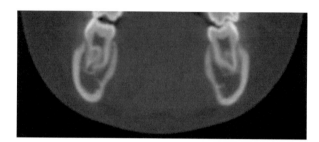

Fig. 7.6 Maxilla after phase 1

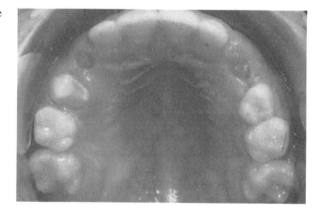

advancements at a time. The basal bone, as seen in the CBCT section view in the lower arch, usually determines the limit for lateral arch development. There can be no stimulus coming from forces upon the lower teeth, which extends enough below the root apices, to develop new bone in that area. On rare occasions the functional space required by the coronoid and mandibular lateral motion can limit the extent of upper arch expansion. The ideal amount of expansion is the amount needed to create the functional space required for normal tongue posture and function. Many orthodontists simply expand enough to coordinate the upper arch to the existing

Fig. 7.7 Mandible after phase 1

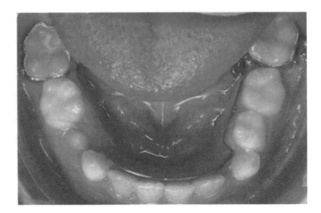

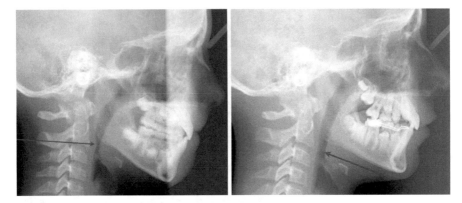

Fig. 7.8 Pretreatment and posttreatment lateral cephalometric X-rays showing increase in AP dimension of the oropharyngeal airway. No tonsils or adenoids were removed in this case

lower arch dimension. This is frequently less stable than more expansion, if the structural changes to the nasal airway aren't enough to create nasal airway patency, along with enough dimension changes to allow for ideal soft tissue function and posture, especially related to the tongue. A new paradigm has been proposed by Steven Olmos for determination of the amount of expansion for pediatric patients with OSA. Rather than using a traditional approach, which is related to creation of adequate space for dental alignment, the goal for expansion should be the dimension that results in the individualized optimum reduction of Apnea-Hypopnea Index (AHI) and Respiratory Effort-Related Arousals (RERA) [38]. Research has shown that myofunctional issues will lead to relapse of expansion and recurrence of sleep apnea in a significant percentage of patients, even when adequate expansion was initially achieved [39]. Myofunctional therapy is a critical part of the treatment needed in many of these skeletally compromised patients with disturbed sleep breathing problems. This will be discussed in greater detail later in this chapter.

In our example case, the upper arch was expanded 9 mm, and the lower arch was laterally developed 7 mm, including uprighting of the posteriors. The patient no longer snores and is no longer a mouth breather at night. The difference in muscle tone associated with his lips is easily seen on these radiographic images. These results have held till the present time (for 6 years). Although a Hyrax was used in this case, almost any expander can be successfully used. Because it can be made to minimize interference with ideal tongue posture and function, a quadhelix made with a lighter wire such as a 0.030″ or 0.032″ is a good choice. Adjustments should be subtle so as to not exceed the rate at which the physiology of the suture and PDL spaces allows for new bony development. Palatal expansion with too great a force risks tearing of the midpalatal suture. As discussed previously, splitting the palate and potentiating fusion across the midpalatal suture seems to be physiologically disadvantageous. Spring expanders seem to function as SME appliances, leaving a viable midpalatal suture.

7.3 Advancing the Entire Maxilla and Developing the Anterior Maxilla, Advancing "A" Point

At times, expansion will not address all the areas of airway constriction or will not create enough oral volume to allow for ideal tongue posture and function. In cases where an area of constriction involves the velopharynx, advancing the entire maxilla can be crucial in improvement of sleep-disordered breathing issues. In the CBCT image from another patient, it can be seen that the area of greatest airway constriction is behind the soft palate, including some adenoidal tissue involvement (Fig. 7.9). Studies have demonstrated that when reverse pull traction appliances are utilized, the entire maxilla is repositioned forward, including PNS [40]. There are several choices when selecting a reverse pull traction appliance. Any such appliance that

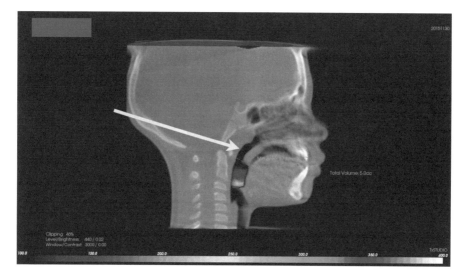

Fig. 7.9 Volumetric airway assessment with CBCT

has a chin cup component will cause the mandible to rotate down and back. This can be advantageous in cases where that is a desired outcome. For cases that have a high angle tendency, a chin cup would lead to an unwanted skeletal change. In general, if there is an oropharyngeal constriction, especially near the level of the chin, rotating the mandible down and back can be problematic. This type of change in mandibular orientation and position has been shown to reposition the hyoid bone down and back [41]. In cases where orthodontic or dentofacial orthopedic treatment has caused the hyoid bone to change orientation and move down and back, a reduction in oropharyngeal airway volume has resulted [42]. Reverse pull appliances that don't have a chin cup include zygomatic masks and Tandem Bow appliances.

Tandem Bow appliances don't place pressure on the forehead, in the region of the prefrontal cortex, and have been shown to successfully advance the maxilla [43]. Tandem Bow appliances can be combined with a palatal expansion appliance to create a fixed upper component for these traction devices. The lower component can be fixed or removable and will have headgear tubes on the buccal in the region of the lower first molars for engagement of a removable bow. Studies have demonstrated that when maxillary protraction appliances are used, a significant increase in upper airway dimensions results [44, 45]. Studies have also demonstrated a significant improvement in AHI in children, as a result of these procedures [45, 46]. An example of mid-face deficiency treated with expansion and a Tandem Bow is shown (Fig. 7.10).

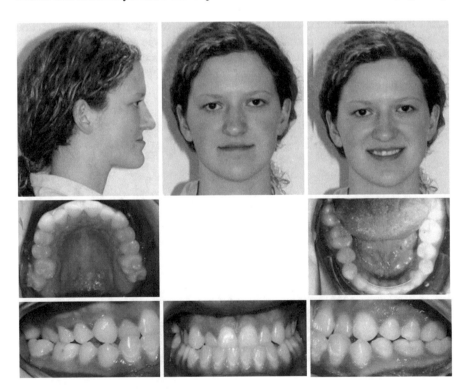

Fig. 7.10 Pretreatment photographs

This is a case that had already been treated in another office, and the patient had presented after having been told that her only option was orthognathic surgery to expand and advance the maxilla. Despite the social pressures associated with entering college, the patient agreed to wear a Tandem Bow appliance for 12 h per day, followed by finishing orthodontic treatment. Her pretreatment lateral ceph is shown below (Fig. 7.11). She is severely midface deficient, with her traced ceph showing a maxillary to mandibular skeletal discrepancy of 17 mm. Fortunately her ANB discrepancy was only 5.6 mm, and it was felt that we could advance her maxilla sufficiently to achieve all needed functional and esthetic goals.

Her tracing and analysis are shown to demonstrate the skeletal problems (Figs. 7.12 and 7.13).

Fig. 7.11 Pretreatment cephalometric X-ray

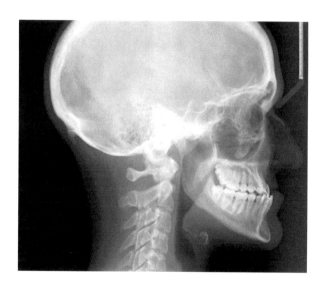

Fig. 7.12 Cephalometric tracing

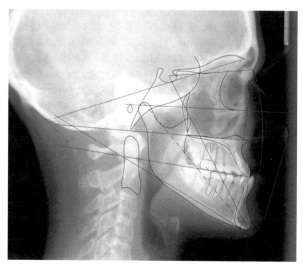

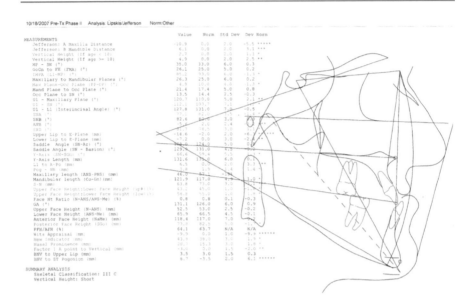

Fig. 7.13 Cephalometric analysis

Treatment was initiated with a Tandem Bow, with a Hyrax expander incorporated into the upper component, as shown below (Fig. 7.14). The patient was very cooperative and the Tandem appliance was worn for 11 months, 12 h per day. It was adjusted to between 250 and 300 g of force per side, totaling 500–600 g total protraction force. Adjustment of the appliance is shown below (Fig. 7.15). Expansion of the Hyrax was accomplished at a rate of 0.5 mm per week until the upper arch had been expanded 11 mm. A US Fisioline Lumix II laser at a bioactive wavelength of 910 nm was used to enhance bony changes and growth [46].

Passive self-ligating (PSL) brackets were then used to enhance bone growth through light forces, which will be discussed below in the further discussion of maxillary advancement. The final results demonstrated a significant advancement of the maxilla and an improvement in the AP dimension of the most restricted aspect of the oropharyngeal airway seen on the lateral cephalometric X-rays (Fig. 7.16). Her final treatment results are shown below, demonstrating a significant improvement in the midface (Fig. 7.17).

This improvement in the mid-face region can be shown to be due to a significant advancement at "A" point of 5.1 mm. In her case, most of this advancement was due to the Tandem Bow appliance, but there was some alignment and advancement through light orthodontic forces using the principles of passive ligation. The pre- and post-overlaid lateral cephalometric tracings show these changes (Fig. 7.18). Her posttreatment records showing the final occlusion are shown below (Fig. 7.19).

Orthodontic advancement of "A" point, using passive self-ligation (PSL), requires a reduction in force levels so that the force of the roots of the upper anteriors on the pressure side of tooth movement into the PDL space doesn't exceed 32 g,

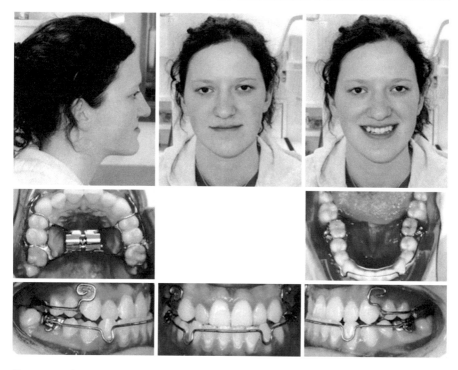

Fig. 7.14 Mid-treatment photographs

Fig. 7.15 Measuring the forward pull at 250–300 g per side

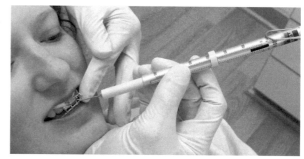

which has been defined as the threshold of applied pressure in order to avoid complete capillary closure in the PDL space [47–49]. Forces at or below this level engender a different mode of tooth movement than forces above it. Traditional orthodontic forces generate a compressive load between 60 and 180 g of force, leading to complete capillary collapse in the periodontal ligament space and an inflammatory response, with cell necrosis in both the PDL space and in the bone, whose vascular supply has been interrupted. At this level of force, teeth can move within existing bone, but other than essentially bone fill in and repair, there is no mechanism to grow bone in advance of a facially moving tooth [48, 49]. When

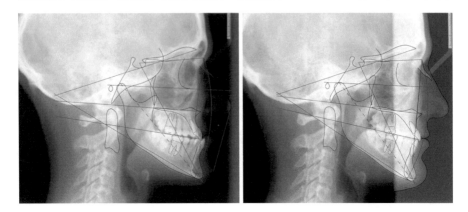

Fig. 7.16 Comparison of pre- (left) and posttreatment lateral cephalometric X-ray

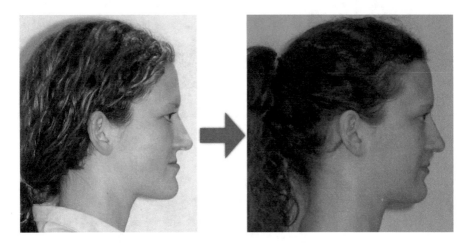

Fig. 7.17 Comparison of pre- (left) and posttreatment

Fig. 7.18 Overlay of pre- and posttreatment cephalometric tracings

Black: Pre-treatment
Green: Post-treatment

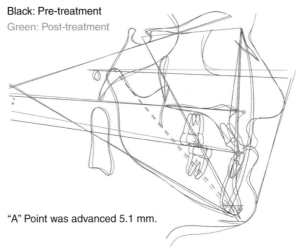

"A" Point was advanced 5.1 mm.

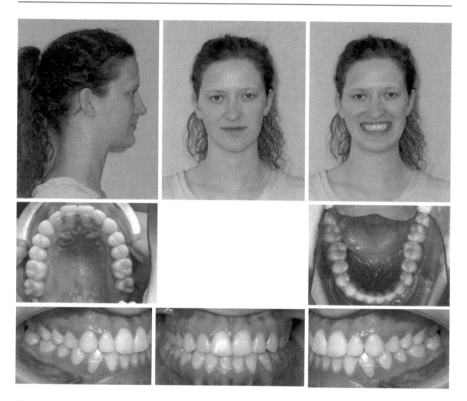

Fig. 7.19 Posttreatment photographs

forces are low enough to not crush the vascular supply in the PDL space, the mechanism of tooth movement and bone remodeling mimics the responses of bone under normal adaptive remodeling or during growth. With consistent light forces, there are piezoelectric forces in response to bone distortion or bending (as there are with heavier forces), but as there is no interruption in blood flow, there is little to no inflammatory response and a very rapid osteoclastic response is fostered. With this osteoclastic response, certain factors are released from the bone by osteoclastic activity. Among the released factors are transforming growth factor beta (TGFβ), which is a cytokine involved in controlling cell growth and differentiation; bone morphometric proteins (BMPs), which are proteins that stimulate bone growth; and insulin-like growth factors I and II (IGF-I and IGF-II), which have growth-regulating functions and also stimulate mitogenic activities. These factors along with released matrix metalloproteinases lead to a coupled response between osteoclasts and osteoblasts, stimulating osteoblastic activity at the bone surface [50]. In this way, as long as force levels are light and inflammation is minimized, new bone can be grown in advance of a facially moving tooth. This principle can be utilized to increase maxillary length and advance "A" point. In mixed dentition, PSL brackets with a light wire that can control torque, as bodily movement of teeth facially is desired, as opposed to tipping, are recommended. The bracketing is a typical mixed dentition 2 × 4 set up, with the primary teeth not bracketed, as shown (Fig. 7.20). A light nickel titanium open coil spring (0.010 × 0.030) is placed from the upper laterals to

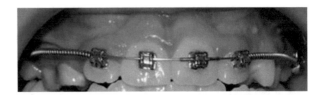

Fig. 7.20 Advancing the upper anterior teeth with fixed mechanics

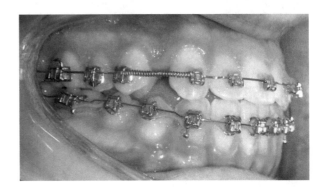

Fig. 7.21 Progress photograph

the upper first molars. The force is carefully measured with a force gauge to not exceed 40 g, as long as there are no spaces between the teeth. This distributes the force so that no tooth exceeds the force that would elicit an inflammatory response and risk moving the tooth out of the bone. If there are spaces, the force is reduced to 30 g until the anteriors are consolidated. For anchorage, a trans-palatal arch (TPA) or fixed expander works well, as in these cases, distalization of the posteriors would be an undesired effect of the spring force. In the permanent dentition, springs are initially placed, with similar force levels, between the upper cuspids and first bicuspids (Fig. 7.21). Torque control is again essential in order to assure stimulation of the bone in front of the upper anterior roots and to avoid excess positive crown torque. Once the anterior teeth have been advanced as far as needed or will not advance further, the springs are moved, and the posteriors are progressively mesialized. Anchorage can be as above or through indirect anchorage using TADs. Once the upper second bicuspids are consolidated forward, the arch is lace tied with steel ligature wire 5 to 5, the upper second molars are disengaged from the arch wire, and the upper molars are brought forward with power chains from the upper second bicuspids to the hooks on the first molar brackets. The second molars will virtually always come forward at the same time. "A" point advancement of approximately 4 mm can be regularly achieved this way. This advancement is promoted and enhanced by the use of a bio-stimulating laser [46]. The most effective laser seems to be the MLS that has a dual wavelength at 808 and 905 nm. Without this laser treatment, the advancement happens, as long as light forces are employed, but to a slightly lesser extent. The laser is also anti-inflammatory, thereby reducing the risk of cortical plate damage and perforation by the roots of the anteriors. An example is shown, from a transfer case presenting mid-treatment, of cortical plate destruction in front of all four upper incisors when advancement was attempted in

Fig. 7.22 Cross-sectional view of anterior teeth

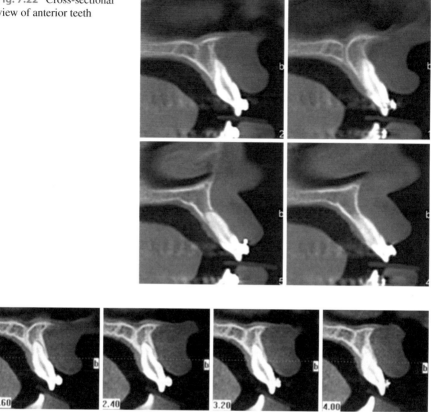

Fig. 7.23 New bone growth as seen on CBCT

another office without using the principles of light forces (Fig. 7.22). The CBCT section view clearly shows that there is essentially no bone remaining in front of the roots of this patient's incisors. Fortunately, we were able to change to PSL brackets and light wires and use light forces, negative root torque, gentle retraction, and the laser to successfully bring these teeth back into the bone. After allowing the bone to mature, we were able to resume treatment, and the anterior teeth and "A" point were advanced ideally for this patient. The CBCT demonstrating new bone in front of the upper incisors is shown (Fig. 7.23).

7.4   Mandibular Advancement

Mandibular advancement using functional appliances is well documented [51–53] and will be mentioned here briefly, as it can be an essential component of airway improvement. As has been discussed above, dentofacial orthopedic or orthodontic procedures that change the position of the mandible have an effect on the position of the hyoid bone. This has the ability to improve the airway if the mandible and hyoid are advanced and has been shown to reduce the airway when retracted or rotated down and back [54]. Mandibular advancement alone has been demonstrated to improve airways and when combined with maxillary development has been shown to have an effect similar to bimaxillary advancement surgery for obstructive sleep apnea [55, 56]. Based on Rabie's research, it seems that when the mandible is advanced incrementally, 3 mm at a time, every 3–4 months, there is a genetic activation at each advancement that speeds and enhances the result [52, 57]. This seems to be true no matter what appliance is used, and as with expansion, technique seems to be more critical than choice of appliance. Maxillary AP position should be corrected before mandibular translation. In order to prohibit any possible maxillary retractive affect from functional appliances, a protraction appliance like a zygomatic facemask may need to be worn at night. When obstruction and airway collapse in OSA is lower in the oropharynx, mandibular advancement can be important in obtaining a successful result.

7.5 Repositioning the Mandible Using a Sibilant Phoneme Registration Protocol/Phonetic Bite to Prevent Upper Airway Collapse

A strategy that has been highly successful for all OSA patients, including pediatric OSA patients, especially in combination with any or all of the appropriate treatments discussed above, is to reposition the mandible using a sibilant phonetic bite registration technique. This bite registration technique has been demonstrated to produce a three-dimensional change in mandibular posture, improving cants, rotations, pitch, and general position to the most achievable, level symmetric posture that skeletal structure allows. It has also been shown that this new mandibular posture opens the airway and reduces airway collapse [58, 59]. This therapy can be accomplished with an orthotic-like removable lower appliance or with composite buildups, usually on the lower deciduous teeth. When used with a removable appliance, it is generally ideal to include an expansion screw as the anterior major connector. With buildups, a lower arch development appliance like a lower "E" expander, as shown above, can easily be incorporated (Figs. 7.23, 7.24, and 7.25). The phonetic bite can be sectioned, and a

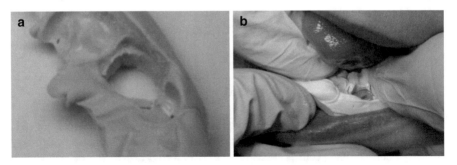

Fig. 7.24 (a) Template for molar "buildup". (b) Template in place

Fig. 7.25 Finished buildup

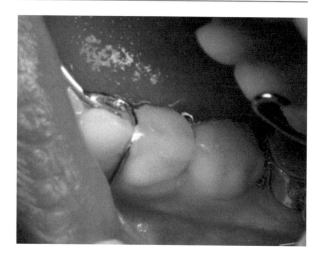

hole can be cut into the bite with a scalpel. This hole can function as a form to build up, to the depth of the bite registration material, the ideal form to hold the registered mandibular posture. This is repeated for at least all four primary lower molars (Fig. 7.24). When the buildups are all in place, the mandibular position mimics the position from the bite registration (Fig. 7.25).

Virtually all of these patients will require palatal expansion to increase oral volume, to improve the nasal airway, and at times to allow for enough space for ideal dental alignment. The ability to laterally develop the lower arch while the upper arch is expanded shortens treatment time and improves airways more quickly. The repositioning of the lower jaw, as described here, can be the most significant procedure in insuring that the patient's airway improvement is maximized.

7.6   Anti-inflammatory Diet and Myofunctional Therapy

Although this chapter is about orthodontic and dentofacial orthopedic strategies to treat pediatric OSA, it would be remiss to not mention what may be the most significant causative factor in creating poor airways, especially poor nasal airways. This factor is an inflammatory dietary intake from the earliest ages. It can be frustrating to expand a nasal airway to a fantastic structural volume that should provide an easily patent airway, only to discover that the high carbohydrate and possibly allergenic diet that the patient consumes has caused the nasal mucosa to become so inflamed that it fills even the increased airway dimension and the airway is still effectively blocked. For many patients, nutritional advice and implementation of an anti-inflammatory diet can be critical in restoring good nasal breathing.

Myofunctional therapy will be discussed later in this chapter, but without normal tongue posture and function, along with normal tone, posture, and function of all the orofacial musculature, the techniques discussed above will be less effective and less stable [39].

7.7 Conclusion

Research has demonstrated that pediatric OSA is essentially a craniofacial structural problem. Causality can have various origins, but without changing the structure, pediatric OSA can only be managed, not cured. The timing for treatment is important, as studies have clearly demonstrated that there is an urgency for intervention, with the likelihood of a permanent negative impact on the entire life of a child with OSA if treatment is delayed, especially if delayed till all the permanent teeth (through the second molars) are erupted.

Full evaluation of all children to be treated is needed in order to determine the points of obstruction and craniofacial anomalies, in order to select the best treatment strategy or combination of strategies that will best correct the issues the child presents with. Treatment of pediatric OSA should always be investigated whenever an orthodontic patient presents for treatment. There is probably no better service that can be accomplished to promote a healthier life for that patient. It also seems that poor airways are significant causes, if not the most primary cause, of malocclusion [1–9, 11–14]; therefore, orthodontic practitioners, as doctors interested in treating their patients to the best possible outcome, should include airway evaluation in their diagnostic protocols.

References

1. Thornval A. Wilhelm Meyer and the adenoids. Arch Otolaryngol. 1969;90:383–6.
2. Pullen HA. Mouth breathing. Dent Cosmos. 1906;48:98–104.
3. M'Kenzie D. Some points of common interest to the rhinologist and the orthodontist. Int J Orthod. 1915;1:9–17.
4. Harvold EP, et al. Primate experiments on oral sensation and dental malocclusion. Am J Orthod. 1973;63:494–508.
5. Harvold EP, et al. Primate experiments on oral respiration. Am J Orthod. 1981;79(4):359–72.
6. Peltomaki T. The effect of mode of breathing on craniofacial growth - revisited. Eur J Orthod. 2007;29(5):426–9.
7. Faria PTM, et al. Dentofacial morphology of mouth breathing. Child Braz Dent J. 2002;13(2):129–32.
8. Bresolin D, et al. Mouth breathing in allergic children: its relationship to dentofacial development. Am J Orthod. 1983;83(4):334–40.
9. Subtelny D. Oral respiration: facial maldevelopment and corrective dentofacial. Orthoped Angle Orthod. 1980;50(3):147–63.
10. Kalha AS. Early orthodontic treatment reduced incisal trauma in children with class II malocclusions. Evid Based Dent. 2014;15(1):18–20.
11. Huang Y, Guilleminault C. Pediatric obstructive sleep apnea and the critical role of oral-facial growth: evidences. Front Neurol Sleep Chronobiol. 2013;3:1–7.
12. Kim JH, et al. The nasomaxillary complex, the mandible, and sleep-disordered breathing. Sleep Breath. 2011;15:185–93.
13. Linder-Aronson A. Their effect on mode of breathing and nasal airflow and their relationship to characteristics of the facial skeleton and the dentition. A biometric, rhino-manometricand cephalometro-radiographic study on children with and without adenoids. Acta Otolaryngol Suppl. 1970;265:1–132.

14. Solow B. Airway adequacy, head posture, and craniofacial morphology. Am J Orthod. 1984;86:214–23.
15. Beebe DW, Gozal D. Obstructive sleep apnea and the prefrontal cortex: towards a comprehensive model linking nocturnal upper airway obstruction to daytime cognitive and behavioral deficits. J Sleep Res. 2002;11:1–16.
16. Gozal D, et al. C-reactive protein, obstructive sleep apnea, and cognitive dysfunction in school-aged children. Am J Respir Crit Care Med. 2007;176:188–93.
17. Carvalho LBC, et al. Cognitive dysfunction in children with sleep-disordered breathing. J Child Neurol. 2005;20(4):400–4.
18. Halbower A, et al, Childhood sleep apnea linked to brain damage, lower IQ. Sci Daily 2006.
19. Halbower A, et al. Childhood obstructive sleep apnea associates with Neuropsychological deficits and neuronal brain injury. PLoS Med. 2006;3(8):1391–402.
20. Young MA. Treatment of obstructive sleep apnea in children. Korean J Pediatr. 2010;53(10):872–9.
21. Suri JC, et al. Outcome of adenotonsillectomy for children with sleep apnea. Sleep Med. 2015;16(10):1181–6.
22. Huang Y, et al. Treatment outcomes of adenotonsillectomy for children with obstructive sleep apnea: a prospective longitudinal study. Sleep. 2014;37(1):71–6.
23. Mitchell RB. Adenotonsillectomy for obstructive sleep apnea in children: outcome evaluated by pre- and postoperative polysomnography. Laryngoscope. 2007;117(10):1844–54.
24. Cistuli P, et al. Treatment of obstructive sleep apnea syndrome by rapid maxillary expansion. Sleep. 1998;21(8):831–5.
25. Giannasi LC, et al. Effect of a rapid maxillary expansion on snoring and sleep in children: a pilot study. Cranio. 2015;33:169.
26. McNamara JA Jr, et al. The role of rapid maxillary expansion in the promotion of oral and general health. Prog Orthod. 2015;16:33.
27. Machado-Junior AJ, et al. Rapid maxillary expansion and obstructive sleep apnea: a review and meta-analysis. Med Oral Patol Cir Bucal. 2016;21:e465. https://doi.org/10.4317/medoral.21073.
28. Guilleminault C, et al. Towards restoration of continuous nasal breathing as the ultimate treatment goal in pediatric obstructive sleep. Apnea Enliven Arch. 2014;1(1):1–5.
29. Linder-Aronson S. Adenoids. Their effect on mode of breathing and nasal airflow and their relationship to characteristics of the facial skeleton and the denition. A biometric, rhino-manometric and cephalometro-radiographic study on children with and without adenoids. Acta Otolaryngol Suppl. 1970;265:1–132.
30. Defabjanis P. Impact of nasal airway obstruction on dentofacial development and sleep disturbances in children: preliminary notes. J Clin Pediatr Dent. 2003;27(2):95–100.
31. Ghoneima A, et al. Accuracy and reliability of cone-beam computed tomography for airway volume analysis. Eur J Orthod. 2011;35:256. https://doi.org/10.1093/ejo/cjr099.
32. Wong CA, et al. Arch dimension changes from successful slow maxillary expansion of unilateral posterior crossbite. Angle Orthod. 2011;81(4):616–22.
33. Zhou Y, et al. Systematic review. The effectiveness of non-surgical maxillary expansion: a meta analysis. Eur J Orthod. 2014;36:233–42.
34. Mobrici P, et al. Slow maxillary expansion in adults: a pilot study. Mondo Ortod. 2012;37(5):7–13.
35. Wehrbein H, et al. The mid-palatal suture in young adults, a radiological-histological investigation. Eur J Orthod. 2001;23:105–14.
36. Herring S, et al. Strain in the braincase and surrounding sutures during function. Am J Phys Anthropol. 2000;112:575–93.
37. Proffit WR. Contemporary orthodontics. 5th ed. St. Louis, MO: Elsevier/Mosby; 2013. p. 537–8. Chapter 14
38. Olmos SR. 3D orthopedic development for pediatric Obstructive Sleep Apnea (OSA). Orthod Pract. 2016;7(2):35–40.

39. Guilleminault C, et al. Critical role of myofascial reeducation in pediatric sleep-disordered breathing. Sleep Med. 2013;14:518–25.
40. Baccetti T, et al. Skeletal effects of early treatment of Class III malocclusion with maxillary expansion and face mask therapy. Am J Orthod Dentofacial Orthop. 1998;113(3):333–43.
41. Ashok KJ, et al. Hyoid bone position in subjects with different vertical jaw dysplasias. Angle Orthod. 2011;81(1):81–5.
42. Wang Q, et al. Changes of pharyngeal airway size and hyoid bone position following orthodontic treatment of Class I bimaxillary protrusion. Angle Orthod. 2012;82(1):115–21.
43. Atalay Z, et al. Dentofacial effects of a modified tandem traction bow appliance. Eur J Orthod. 2010;32:655–61.
44. Gupta R, et al. An evaluation of the sagittal upper airway dimension changes following treatment with maxillary protraction appliances. Int J Contemp Dent. 2011;2(5):59–65.
45. Peanchitlertkajorn S. RPE and orthodontic protraction facemask as an alternative therapy for severe obstructive sleep apnea associated with maxillary hypoplasia. J Dental Sleep Med. 2016;3(1):33–4.
46. Martinasso G, et al. Effect of superpulsed laser irradiation on bone formation in a human osteoblast-like cell line. Minerva Stomatol. 2007;56(1-2):27–30.
47. Schwarz AM. Tissue changes incident to orthodontic tooth movement. Int J Orthod. 1932;18:331–52.
48. Meeran NA. Biological response at the cellular level within the periodontal ligament on application of orthodontic force – an update. J Orthod Sci. 2012;1(1):2–10.
49. Krishnan V, Davidovitch Z. Biological mechanisms of tooth movement. London: Wiley-Blackwell; 2009. p. 180–4. Chapter 10
50. Hill PA. Bone remodeling. Br J Orthod. 1998;25:101–7.
51. Voudouris JC, et al. Improved clinical use of twin-block and Herbst as a result of radiating viscoelastic tissue forces on the condyle and fossa in treatment and long term retention: Growth relativity. AJODO. 2000;117:247–66.
52. Rabie ABM, et al. Functional appliance therapy accelerates and anhances condylar growth. AJODO. 2003;123:40–8.
53. Pancherz H, et al. The Herbst appliance: research-based updated clinical possibilities. World J Orthod. 2000;1:17–31.
54. Schütz B, et al. Class II correction improves nocturnal breathing in adolescents. Angle Orthod. 2011;81(2):222–8.
55. Cobo Plana J. Orthodontics and the upper airway. Orthod Fr. 2004;75(1):31–7.
56. Ibitayo AO, et al. Dentoskeletal effects of functional appliances vs bimaxillary surgery in hyperdivergent Class II patients. Angle Orthod. 2011;81(2):304–11.
57. Wey MC, et al. Stepwise advancement versus maximum jumping with headgear activator. Eur J Orthod. 2007;29:283–93.
58. Singh DG, Olmos SR. Use of a sibilant phoneme registration protocol to prevent upper airway collapse in patients with TMD. Sleep Breath. 2007;11:209. https://doi.org/10.1007/s11325-007-0104-3.
59. Mahony D, Lipskis EA. Bite registration and OSA appliances: the phonetic bite and the Moses bite. Aust Dent Pract. 2012:56–60.

Treatment of Myofunctional Pathology

8

Joy L. Moeller, Martha Macaluso, and Ruth Marsiliani

8.1   What Is Myofunctional Therapy

Myofunctional therapy is the neurologic reeducation of the orofacial muscles. It is a rehabilitation therapy program designed to re-pattern stomatognathic functions, such as chewing, swallowing, and breathing. This is accomplished through the use of therapeutic techniques and positive behavioral modification [1, 2]. The therapy allows the brain to develop new neural pathways through repetition, time, and experience. Once the new behavior is learned and adopted, those neural connections are reinforced. This creates a more permanent neural change commonly known as neuroplasticity. Repetition of the therapeutic techniques will help to increase the strength, tone, and coordination of the stomatognathic muscles and help to develop facial symmetry. The purposes of these exercises are to:

- Recover and improve dyskinetic muscle function.
- Restore deficient muscle tone.
- Reacquire correct posture (tongue, jaw, and lips).
- Reeducate functions (swallowing, chewing, and breathing).
- Reduce and eliminate habits such as thumb sucking, pacifier use, nail biting, lip or hair sucking or biting, tongue sucking, leaning, and others.

J. L. Moeller (✉)
Academy of Orofacial Myofunctional Therapy, Pacific Palisades, CA, USA

M. Macaluso
Academy of Orofacial Myofunctional Therapy, Pacific Palisades, CA, USA

New York University College of Dentistry, New York, NY, USA

R. Marsiliani
Academy of Orofacial Myofunctional Therapy, Pacific Palisades, CA, USA

New York University College of Dentistry, New York, NY, USA

The City University of New York, New York City College of Technology, Brooklyn, NY, USA

© Springer Nature Switzerland AG 2019
E. Liem (ed.), *Sleep Disorders in Pediatric Dentistry*,
https://doi.org/10.1007/978-3-030-13269-9_8

Awareness and elimination of oral habits must be addressed conjointly with myofunctional disorders, or they may affect the fluidity and process of the therapy.

In the United States, breathing re-education is incorporated along with chewing and proper swallowing, to assist in the treatment of myofunctional disorders. Breathing education looks at nasal breathing versus mouth breathing; the volume of air taken in during inhalation, and the muscles recruited during breathing (movement of the diaphragm). Both oral habit elimination and breathing education are important for continued positive progression and desired outcome of the therapy. Additionally, to achieve optimum results, myofunctional therapists work collaboratively with ENTs, allergists, and orthodontists.

8.2   Importance of Myofunctional Therapy

Myofunctional therapy for the treatment of myofunctional disorders has demonstrated to be an important adjunct in the treatment of (sleep) breathing disorders, orthodontic treatment, temporal mandibular joint dysfunction (TMD), masticatory dysfunctions, and digestive and postural problems [2–7].

Myofunctional therapy also addresses underlying issues pertaining to various health-related disorders, and therefore aides in the reduction of general healthcare costs.

Myofunctional therapy can aid in the restoration of continuous nasal breathing, and if implemented during the early years of development, it can positively affect craniofacial growth deficits associated with sleep-disordered breathing [2, 8–10]. Currently, clinical studies have proposed breathing education as a necessary adjunctive therapy in the treatment of sleep-disordered breathing [8, 11].

Part of the therapeutic breathing techniques include:

1. Correct use of breathing muscles
2. Reducing or normalizing the correct volume of air
3. Timing the therapy at rest, during activity, speech, sleep, and sport

Adenotonsillectomy is often prescribed in children to improve airway patency and symptoms associated with sleep apnea [10–13]. However, a child who has suffered from enlarged tonsils and adenoids may have ingrained habits such as; mouth breathing, poor oral rest posture, and improper breathing patterns [8, 11]. These perpetuating habits, if not corrected, can promote relapse of obstruction and affect proper orofacial growth [8, 11]. For that reason, myofunctional therapy should be incorporated into the protocols following the adenotonsillectomy; myofunctional therapy should be performed after the surgical procedure in order to create proper oral rest posture and promote nasal breathing [10, 11, 13].

The rehabilitation process of the orofacial and oropharyngeal muscle groups, create adequate airway patency [2, 3]. A meta-analysis conducted by Camacho et al. demonstrated a decrease in the frequency of apneas measured by the Apnea Hypopnea Index (AHI). Children's AHI decreased by 62% and for adults by 50% after going through myofunctional therapy [13].

8.3   Etiology of Orofacial Myofunctional Disorders

Orofacial myofunctional disorders (OMDs) are a group of various stomatognathic functional disorders; it can affect directly or indirectly: dental occlusion, stability of outcome of orthodontic treatment, stability of periodontal therapy, temporomandibular joint functions, facial esthetic, facial skeletal growth, pharyngeal airway dimension, and speech [1].

The etiological origin of OMDs is multifactorial, and it is difficult to isolate a single factor. Some causative factors include but are not limited to:

- Noxious oral habits (thumb sucking, nail biting, etc.)
- Bottle feeding, baby food leading to incorrect chewing/swallowing
- Pacifier and spouted sippy cup overuse
- Structural airway restriction
- Restricted or altered oral tissues (tongue and lip ties)
- Enlarged tonsils/adenoids
- Craniofacial development (underdevelopment of maxilla and mandible)
- Facial asymmetry

8.4   Assessment of Myofunctional Disorders

Professionals who work with myofunctional disorders have different tools available for assessment, based on their needs, scope of practice, and preferences. Myofunctional therapists, being a multidisciplinary group, use various tools and practices, which often overlap but retain some individual characteristics depending on the background of the therapist. Moreover, myofunctional therapists are better trained to identify some concurrent signs and symptoms of sleep breathing disorders which then allow the proper referral along with education of patient and caregivers (in the case of children) and treatment of the underlying orofacial functions, which are either affected or are a contributing factor in sleep disorders.

Assessments may include:

1. Mouth versus nasal breathing
2. Low and forward tongue rest posture
3. Tongue thrusts
4. Noxious oral habits
5. Forward head posture
6. Overdeveloped mentalis muscle
7. Facial grimace
8. Lack of lip seal
9. Swallowing and chewing
10. Restricted frenulums: labial, buccal, and lingual
11. Palate width
12. Mallampati or Friedman score

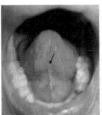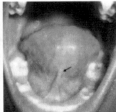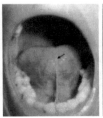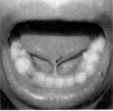

Fig. 8.1 Photos of restricted frenulums selectively chosen from the "Lingual Frenulum Protocol with Scores for Children-Adults" demonstrating varying degrees of lingual frenulum restrictions (with permission from I. Marchesan Lingual Frenum Protocol 2014)

13. Dental open bites
14. Scalloped tongue
15. Tongue strength

Assessment protocols, such as the Orofacial Myofunctional Evaluation Protocol with Scores (OMES) [14] or the Orofacial Myofunctional Evaluation with Scores (MBGR) [15], have been validated and are important tools for a complete evaluation. Using validated protocols, such as those of Roberta Martinelli, Irene Marchesan, and Allison Hazelbaker, is essential for the evaluation of altered oral tissues. These protocols will help to assess altered oral tissues like the labial and lingual frenulum restrictions (Fig. 8.1), which are essential to determine if a frenectomy should be performed.

Therapeutic techniques and post-op wound healing techniques with a myofunctional therapist are essential to maximize the benefits of the frenulum release, including labial, lingual, and buccal restrictions [9, 16, 17].

8.5   Who Does Myofunctional Therapy?

Many healthcare professions from various countries adopt myofunctional principals within the scope of their practice. In Japan most myofunctional therapists are dental hygienists, in Brazil most are speech pathologists, while in some other countries, they are primarily physical therapists. In the United States, speech pathologists, dental hygienists, physical therapists, and occupational therapists are the primary providers of the therapy. In all cases an additional postgraduate training is required.

8.6   Treatment of Myofunctional Disorders

Treatments of myofunctional disorders include isolating and activating muscles in the head and neck and re-patterning them to optimize proper function. Myofunctional therapists generally work with a team of healthcare workers; commonly they work alongside dentists, orthodontists, medical doctors, and speech therapists.

Myofunctional therapy is a therapeutic program by which problems of articulation are often improved because the patients have better control of their muscle functions and tongue placement [17]. There are eight intrinsic and extrinsic muscles of the tongue, which need to work independently and interdependently in order to articulate sounds and swallow correctly.

As an example, myofunctional therapists begin with training the tongue to rest up on the palate. One way this is accomplished is by having the patient hold an orthodontic elastic rubber band to the roof of the mouth with the tongue, for a specific period of time with the lips together. During the same appointment, the patient will use different strings, buttons, and chewing devices; in order to activate and strengthen, or relax some of the muscles of mastication and the perioral muscles.

Proper symmetrical chewing, gathering the food in the middle of the tongue, and swallowing without the assistance of the perioral muscles are very important parts of myofunctional treatment. Bilateral chewing has been shown to help with TMD issues [4, 5].

The therapy is progressive, whereby the exercises are sequential and become more advanced. Certain exercises are repeated depending on the needs of the patient, while focusing on the goals of therapy. The therapy program is usually done over a period of 1 year to attain long-term retention of the results. Myofunctional therapists work on enhancing proper chewing, breathing, swallowing, and functional posturing while eliminating oral habits that interfere with this process.

8.7   Patients with Sleep Disorders

The meta-analysis previously mentioned demonstrated a reduction in AHI by 50% in adults and 62% in children, in patients treated for sleep apnea with myofunctional therapy [13]. Recent studies reveal how myofunctional therapy in conjunction with Continuous Positive Airway Pressure (CPAP) demonstrates better adherence and results [18]. Furthermore, the Mandibular Advancement Device (MAD) and Oral Appliance Therapy (OAT) may be more comfortable with myofunctional therapy [4, 5]. The stretching and developing of facial symmetry with specific exercises will assure better compliance for the patient, and the dentist will be able to deliver the best results possible.

Snoring may be one of the first signs of sleep apnea. We now have studies demonstrating myofunctional therapy as an effective measure to eliminate snoring. The tightening and toning of the pharyngeal muscles, soft palate and uvula, can be accomplished through neuromuscular repatterning that will prevent, minimize, or eliminate snoring [19].

It has been hypothesized in many studies that nocturnal bruxism may be a sign of a compromised airway, TMD, or sleep apnea [20]. Research can confirm that myofunctional therapy will help to decrease pain intensity and lower bruxism episodes with statistically significant results [20].

The tongue has both intrinsic and extrinsic muscles. The extrinsic muscles, if not patterned correctly, may affect breathing, posture, and neck discomfort. Especially for patients with sleep apnea, myofunctional therapists work closely to activate and isolate the genioglossus muscle or the base of the tongue, which if it is not working correctly may occlude the airway. The pharyngeal muscles need to be toned and restored to normal function, which by certain throat and back of the tongue exercises may make a huge difference over time. An example would be to bite on a pediatric bite block, make a "K" sound three times with the bite block in, and swallow lifting the back of the tongue. Repeat this six times three times a day.

8.8 Prevention with Early Intervention

Early intervention and prevention should begin in the womb. The expectant mother should be educated prior to the third semester of pregnancy. During this time the expectant mother experiences challenges in weight gain and times of stress that affect breathing regulation and volume, which can onset mouth breathing.

Bottle feeding, baby foods, and pacifiers need to be redesigned to promote airway patency of the growing infant. More emphasis needs to be on promoting the development of a wider palate earlier and preventing its collapse. In cases where infants eat smooth foods, the infant learns not to masticate. Consequently, proper chewing may never develop causing the muscles associated with the airway to collapse. Also, not digesting their food properly occurs with a lack of chewing and may lead to aerophagia.

Restricted lingual, labial, and buccal frenulums need to be released earlier and checked for the need of possible revisions. These restricted oral tissues can lead to relapse of orthodontic and orthognathic surgical results. Recent studies demonstrate how these restrictions may also lead to sleep breathing disorders [9, 16].

8.9 Summary

Myofunctional therapy is a neurologic reeducation program which uses repetition, time, and experience to initiate neural changes known as neuroplasticity. Although it is not a novel treatment, it has re-emerged its saliency with the advent of sleep apnea. Myofunctional therapy treats OMDs such as (sleep) breathing disorders, orthodontic treatment (Fig. 8.2), temporal mandibular joint dysfunction, masticatory disorders,

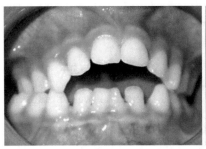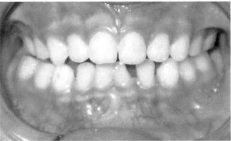

Fig. 8.2 Before (left) and after (right) myofunctional therapy

and digestive and postural problems. The etiological origin of OMDs is multifactorial, and it is difficult to isolate a single factor. Specialized training allows myofunctional therapists to identify signs and symptoms associated with OMDs, which may seem ubiquitous. Important tools are available that will facilitate a complete and comprehensive evaluation. Ultimately, the goal of this therapy is to increase the strength, tone, and coordination of the stomatognathic muscles, help to develop facial symmetry, create proper oral rest posture, and promote nasal breathing.

In recent years, myofunctional therapy has gained more validity as researchers incorporate myofunctional therapy into their studies across the disciplines. We hope that this therapy will soon be incorporated into the protocols following the adenotonsillectomy and considered as another alternative for the treatment of sleep apnea. Today we see the evolution of myofunctional therapy as it pertains to the treatment of sleep apnea. It is being applied in conjunction with CPAP, MAD, and OAT demonstrating enhanced treatment outcomes and adherence, which is critical for the well-being of the patient.

Myofunctional therapists generally work with a team. They include dentists, orthodontists, medical doctors, and speech therapists. Prevention of myofunctional disorders may be possible now through early intervention with therapeutic techniques that have been used in pediatric dentistry, speech therapy, and orthodontics for many years. More research is needed in this area, but preliminary studies are supporting the value of changing the *function* as well as the *structure* in order to successfully treat and prevent many disorders. The team approach is the most important and most beneficial avenue for the patient's health and well-being.

References

1. Paskay LC. OMD orofacial myofunctional disorders: assessment, prevention and treatment. J Appl Oral Sci. 2012:34–40.
2. Moeller JL, Paskay LC, Gelb ML. Myofunctional therapy: a novel treatment of pediatric sleep-disordered breathing. Sleep Med Clin. 2014;9:235.
3. Sugawara Y, Ishihara Y, Takano-Yamamoto T, Yamashiro T, Kamioka H. Orthodontic treatment of a patient with unilateral orofacial muscle dysfunction: the efficacy of myofunctional therapy on the treatment outcome. Am J Orthod Dentofacial Orthop. 2016;150(1):167–80. https://doi.org/10.1016/j.ajodo.2015.08.021.
4. Felício CM, Melchior MD, Da Silva MAMR. Effects of orofacial myofunctional therapy on temporomandibular disorders. Cranio. 2010;28(4):249–59. https://doi.org/10.1179/crn.2010.033.
5. Machado BC, Mazzetto MO, Antonio M, Da Silva MR, Felício CM. Effects of oral motor exercises and laser therapy on chronic temporomandibular disorders: a randomized study with follow-up. Lasers Med Sci. 2016;31(5):945–54. https://doi.org/10.1007/s10103-016-1935-6.
6. Boyd KL, Sheldon SH. Childhood sleep disordered breathing: a dental perspective. In: Principles and practice of pediatric sleep medicine. Philadelphia, PA: Elsevier; 2013. Chapter 34.
7. Maffei C, et al. Orthodontic intervention combined with myofunctional therapy increases electromyographic activity of masticatory muscles in patients with skeletal unilateral posterior crossbite. Acta Odontol Scand. 2014;72:298.
8. Guilleminault C, Sullivan SS. Towards restoration of continuous nasal breathing as the ultimate treatment goal in pediatric obstructive sleep apnea. enliven: pediatrics and neonatal biology enliven. Pediatr Neonatal Biol. 2014;01(01):1. https://doi.org/10.18650/2379-5824.11001.

9. Huang YS, et al. Short lingual frenulum and obstructive sleep apnea in children. Int J Pediatr Res. 2015;1:1.
10. Villa MP, Brasili L, Ferretti A, Vitelli O, Rabasco J, Mazzotta AR, Martella S. Oropharyngeal exercises to reduce symptoms of OSA after AT. Sleep Breath. 2014;19(1):281–9. https://doi.org/10.1007/s11325-014-1011-z.
11. Seo-Young L, Guilleminault C, et al. Mouth breathing, "nasal disuse," and pediatric sleep-disordered breathing. Sleep Breath. 2015;19(4):1257–64.
12. Villa MP, Brasili L, Ferretti A, Vitelli O, Rabasco J, Mazzotta AR, Pietropaoli N, Martella S. Oropharyngeal exercises to reduce symptoms of OSA after AT. Sleep Breath. 2014;19(1):281–9.
13. Camacho M, Certal V, et al. Myofunctional therapy to treat obstructive sleep apnea: a systematic review and meta-analysis. Sleep. 2015;38(5):669–75.
14. Felicio OM, Ferreira CL. Protocol of orofacial myofunctional evaluation with scores. IntJ Pediatr Otorhinolaryngol. 2008;72(3):367–75.
15. Marchesan IQ, Berrentin-Felix G, Genaro KF. MBGR protocol of orofacial myofunctional evaluation with scores. Int J Orofacail Myol. 2012;38:38–77.
16. Olivi G, Signore A, Olivi M. Genovese: lingual frenectomy: functional evaluation and new therapeutical approach. Eur J Paediatr Dent. 2012;13(2):101.
17. Hazelbaker A. Tongue tie: morphogenesis, impact, assessment, and treatment. Columbus, OH: Aiden and Eva Press Books; 2010.
18. Diafária G, Santos-Silva R, Truksinas E, et al. Myofunctional therapy improves adherence to continuous positive airway pressure treatment. Sleep Breath. 2017;21:387. https://doi.org/10.1007/s11325-016-1429-6.
19. Camacho M, Guilleminault C, Wei JM, et al. Oropharyngeal and tongue exercises (myofunctional therapy) for snoring: a systematic review and meta-analysis. Eur Arch Otorhinolaryngol. 2018;275:849. https://doi.org/10.1007/s00405-017-4848-5.
20. Klasser GD, Balasubramaniam R. Sleep bruxism: what orthodontists need to know? In: Kandasamy S, Greene C, Rinchuse D, Stockstill J, editors. TMD and orthodontics. Cham: Springer; 2015.

Future Perspectives of Sleep Disorder Treatment in Pediatric Dentistry

9

Edmund Liem

Pediatric sleep breathing disorders (SBD) deserve attention, because it is associated with significant morbidity, potentially impacting on long-term neurocognitive and behavioral development, as well as cardiovascular outcomes and metabolic homeostasis during a critical phase of formative years. The presence of low-grade systemic inflammation and increased oxidative stress seen in this condition is believed to underpin the development of these OSA-related morbidities. Pediatric SDB deserves specific attention by those who are positioned best to screen and detect signs and symptoms of pediatric sleep breathing disorders. General dentists happen to be in that position!

General dentists do see children from the age of 2 or earlier on a regular base; what they lack currently are the skills and knowledge to recognize the signs and symptoms of pediatric OSA. This topic is at this time not in the curriculum of dental schools worldwide, and it might be years away before this will happen. Therefore this is the time to start learning and be engaged in pediatric sleep breathing disorders. Some dentists are already treating adults with OSA (obstructive sleep apnea), and they soon realized that the treatment they provide is a lifelong treatment/management. Treating children diagnosed with SBD has a different dimension; it has the potential of preventing or *eliminating* the breathing disorder, a condition that affects not only physical, mental and metabolic condition of the patient but also the neurocognitive development of the child.

In this book you have seen that screening, testing, diagnosis, management, and treatment requires a multidisciplinary approach. Every discipline plays a role, and everybody needs to communicate with each other. We have also seen that several approaches exist and all of them are complementary to each other. Most of them are not interchangeable, but complimentary. Myofunctional therapy on its own might not do the trick; orthodontics on its own might also not be optimal, but together they could be very powerful.

E. Liem (✉)
Vancouver TMJ and Sleep Therapy Centre, Burnaby, BC, Canada

© Springer Nature Switzerland AG 2019
E. Liem (ed.), *Sleep Disorders in Pediatric Dentistry*,
https://doi.org/10.1007/978-3-030-13269-9_9

Treating children who are already been diagnosed with OSA is one good approach; however, preventing and providing early treatment of SDB is one whole step ahead, and this is where the future lies.

Dr. Christian Guilleminault, the universally most respected expert in pediatric OSA, said this: "Restoration of Continuous Nasal Breathing as the Ultimate Treatment Goal in Pediatric Obstructive Sleep Apnea" [1].

What this means is that without restoring nasal breathing, you have not addressed a fundamental cause of OSA or SBD. All treatment approaches should have this as ultimate goal, no matter if the approach is preventive, conservative, nonsurgical, or even surgical. Crudely and over-simplified said, the nose is for breathing; the mouth is for drinking and eating. Breathing through the mouth should be considered as an emergency option. When the nose is blocked for whatever reason, it is fortunate that we can breathe through the mouth; however continuous habitual breathing through the mouth (Fig. 9.1) will lead to many issues as described and discussed in Chapters 3–8.

You may have noticed that in this book there is no separate chapter dedicated to tonsil and/or adenoidectomy. You can find a brief discussion in Chapter 1. This omission is done on purpose. Tonsil and/or adenoidectomy (T&A) is still considered by many as the first-line option in treatment of pediatric OSA; however more and

Fig. 9.1 Child with retrognathia and mouth breathing

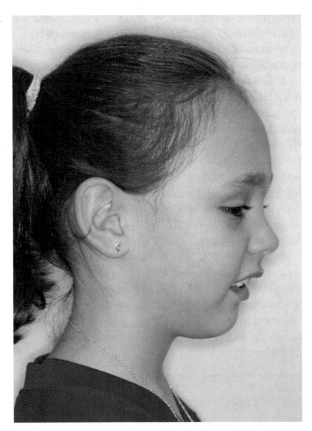

more publications are showing a poor outcome with 50–70% unresolved or recurrent OSA. Guilleminault et al. (2004) demonstrated complete resolution of OSA following adenotonsillectomy in only 51% of non-obese prepubertal children [1, 2]. More and more data are supporting that T&A is of limited value for long-term treatment of pediatric SDB. It still has value as an emergency (first-line, short-term) intervention approach to pediatric SDB. More research needs to be done to understand the cause of enlargement of these lymphatic tissues and how to prevent them.

As the astute reader has found, in this final chapter and throughout this book, the terms SBD (sleep breathing disorder) and OSA (obstructive sleep apnea) are being used. There is another acronym that is often being used: SDB (sleep disordered breathing); currently there is no *official* difference between the three acronyms (some will disagree with this statement), and they seem to be used interchangeably. In this context it is good to introduce another term that is related to this topic: Upper Airway Resistance Syndrome (UARS). At first glance this is a similar condition; however there are some key differences. In simple terms, sleep-test data shows that UARS, the apneas and hypopneas are either absent or very low in patients with UARS. UARS does cause arousals and sleep fragmentation but can be as detrimental as OSA for the child. The problem at this time is that UARS is difficult to diagnose, even with a full polysomnogram (PSG). It is often missed in classical polysomnographic diagnostic approaches and misdiagnosed as simple snoring or idiopathic hypersomnia and thereby is often left (mistakenly) untreated.

There is also no chapter about positive airway pressure (PAP) for pediatric SDB; this modality could be in many cases live-saving; however, the idea of a life-long continuous wear (during sleep) of a PAP unit is abhorrent. A PAP treatment is highly effective by opening the collapsible portion of the airway; however the long-term wear by growing children comes with side effects of potential stunning the craniofacial growth and thus stunning the bony structures where the airway muscles are attached. At 6 years of age, the human head has reached about 60% of an adult, and if the craniofacial growth is stunned, the implication for airway size could be longterm. The issue is that the interface mask needed to deliver the positive airway pressure is putting a pressure in the midface, and this inhibits the craniofacial growth, especially the nasomaxillary complex. The sooner the child is treated with a different modality that enhances craniofacial growth, the better the long-term outcome most likely will be. Excellent sample cases of these types of orthopedic treatments (orthotropic, or correct growth guidance) can be found at the end of Chapter 4.

Many questions exist about the role of orthodontics in prevention and treatment of pediatric or even adult SDB or OSA. There are many heated debates around this controversial topic. Inside this heated discussion, there are many opinions about any airway relationship between orthodontic with premolar extractions and without. Does premolar extraction affect the airway and contribute to (the development of) SDB, OSA, or UARS? Larsen et al. (2015) published an article where they concluded that *extraction orthodontic treatment is not supported as a significant factor in the cause of OSA*. In this article they extracted large amount of (*n* = 584) data from an electronic health record from an insurance company and compared cases where premolars were extracted or not, and after matching gender and BMI (body

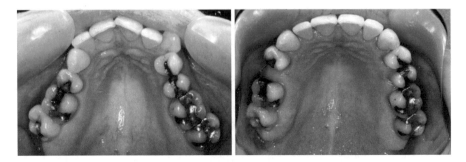

Fig. 9.2 Left: Pretreatment upper jaw with one right premolar removed; very narrow, collapsed maxilla, resulting in a small tongue space. Right: (Same patient) Posttreatment upper jaw with space re-opened where the premolar previously was extracted; resulting in much larger tongue space

mass index), they concluded: *The prevalence of OSA was not significantly different between the groups (OR = 1.14, p = 0.144)* [3].

There are many critics on this study; one of them is there is also no data on age of onset, comorbidities, or severity or type of sleep-disordered breathing. While they probably couldn't get all of that data for the whole cohort, they should have been able to get at least the last 5–10 years worth, which would have added to the study. It would have been very relevant to know which group had more severe indices of disease and should have been possible given their access to medical insurance data. This debate will continue for the meantime without a clear-cut conclusion.

Using common logic, one can make a hard conclusion that the oral volume is different in size for cases where (premolar) extractions are done compared to those non-extraction cases. The oral volume in extraction cases is for sure *not larger* than the non-extraction cases. This is where the tongue resides, and we know that tongue position plays a crucial role in oral volume, airway resistance, and airflow. You be the judge! (Fig. 9.2).

9.1   Ankyloglossia

Dr. Christian Guilleminault from Stanford University mentioned that short lingual frenulum is a frequent phenotype for pediatric sleep apnea [4].

Quite often the finding of a short lingual frenulum is triggered by difficulties with breastfeeding (newborn infants) or at school with some speech impediments. However most of the time, there is no lingual frenulum inspection done, and the children are taught to learn to "deal" (= adapt) with it. Speech pathologists are not always trained to diagnose short lingual frenulum (Fig. 9.3) nor do they have the tools to screen for pediatric OSA. Chapter 8 has a section about short lingual frenum.

A short lingual frenulum can cause difficulties in sucking, swallowing, and speech. The altered (adapted) tongue functions caused by a short lingual frenulum can lead to a non-optimal craniofacial growth [4], which decreases the size of upper airway support leading to a smaller airway and as such increases the risk of upper airway collapsibility during sleep. Treatment for a short lingual frenulum (commonly called

Fig. 9.3 Short lingual frenulum

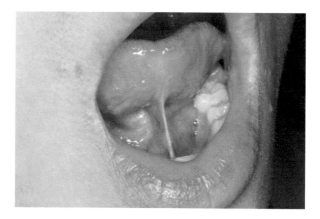

"tongue-tie") consists of surgically releasing the connective tissue that connects the floor of the mouth and the tongue base. This can be done with scalpel, scissors, or laser, and each method has its benefits and limitations. In the past lingual frenectomy has often failed due to frequent re-attachments; optimal result can be achieved by following a protocol that includes specific pre- and post-surgery myofunctional exercises. Due to limitation of space, this topic is not further discussed in detail in this book.

9.2 Premature Births [5–6]

According to Yu-Shu Huang and Christian Guilleminault et al., premature infants have more sleep problems than full-term infants, including the known risk of abnormal breathing during sleep. Dr. Guilleminault says: During the last trimester of pregnancy there is a continuous training of the sucking-swallow reflex with absorption of 1 cm^3 of amniotic fluid initially to 500 cm^3 just before birth. This "training" is missed by those who are born prematurely. The study of premature infants has shown that the more premature the infant, the more health problems are present, and there is a clear impact of the absence of complete training with premature birth: The size of the oral cavity is abnormally small, and muscles are hypotonic, in particular those involved in upper airway and facial functions. This in part does not lead to a normal craniofacial growth and could lead to mouth breathing and incorrect tongue posture and smaller airway that is more prone to collapse during sleep. We have to remember that 60% of the growth of the skull happens before the age of 6. This is a critical time for observation and if needed intervention. With the right education and interest, a general dentist happens to be at the right position to observe properly the signs and symptoms of pediatric OSA.

9.3 Conclusion

Pediatric OSA in non obese children is a disorder of oral-facial growth [2]. This quote from Dr. Christian Guilleminault embodies the unique role that dentistry, including orthodontics and dentofacial orthopedic, has in the prevention and treatment of pediatric OSA. Dentistry is the only discipline that can promote proper craniofacial growth in the midfacial area by non surgical methods.Most dentist and orthodontist are not aware of this role and it is time to start learning how to recognize the signs and symptoms of pediatric OSA. And for those who wants to participate in treatment of these children, it is time to explore the many options dentofacial orthopedics, orthodontics and myofunctional therapy can offer to promote optimal oral-facial growth. Once you have learned the medical side of pediatric OSA (Chapters 1 and 2), you will be able to participate and contribute to the treatment of pediatric OSA. There are many techniques available and this book will be helpful to give the dentist a solid foundation in finding what works for them. When choosing a technique, keep in mind that it must be suitable in primary and mixed dentition. Waiting till all primary teeth are exfoliated (age 9–12) as it is commonly done with traditional orthodontics, is far too late if you would like to have a positive effect on craniofacial growth. Please note that there are more techniques out there that are not discussed in this book (e.g. ALF, Myobrace). All techniques must have as ultimate treatment goal, as stated by Dr. Christian Guilleminault: Restoration of Continuous Nasal Breathing [1].

References

1. Guilleminault C, Sullivan SS. Pediatr Neonatol Biol. 2014;1(1):001.
2. Huang Y-S, Guilleminault C. Pediatric obstructive sleep apnea and the critical role of oral-facial growth: evidences. Front Neurol. 2012;3:184.
3. Larsen AJ, et al. Evidence supports no relationship between obstructive sleep apnea and premolar extraction: an electronic health records review. J Clin Sleep Med. 2015;11(12):1443–8. https://doi.org/10.5664/jcsm.5284.
4. Guilleminault C. A frequent phenotype for paediatric sleep apnoea: short lingual frenulum. ERJ Open Res. 2016;2(3):00043-2016.
5. Huang Y-S, Paiva T, Hsu J-F, Kuo M-C, Guilleminault C. Sleep and breathing in premature infants at 6 months post-natal age. Front Neurol. 2013;3:184.
6. Sharma PB, Baroody F, Gozal D, Lester LA. Obstructive sleep apnea in the formerly preterm infant: an overlooked diagnosis. Front Neurol. 2011;2:73.

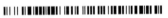

Printed in the United States
By Bookmasters